Urology Inst
A Comprehe

Urology Instrumentation
A Comprehensive Guide

Editors

Ravindra B Sabnis MS MCh
Chairman
Department of Urology
Muljibhai Patel Urological Hospital
Nadiad, Gujarat, India

Sujata K Patwardhan MS MCh
Professor and Head
Department of Urology
Seth GS Medical College and KEM Hospital
Mumbai, Maharashtra, India

Arvind P Ganpule MS DNB MNAMS
Vice-Chairman
Department of Urology
Muljibhai Patel Urological Hospital
Nadiad, Gujarat, India

Assistant Editors

Amit S Bhattu MS DNB
Fellow in Endourology and Laparo-robotic Urology
Consultant Urologist
Muljibhai Patel Urological Hospital
Nadiad, Gujarat, India

Abhishek G Singh MS MCh DNB
Consultant Urologist
Muljibhai Patel Urological Hospital
Nadiad, Gujarat, India

JAYPEE *The Health Sciences Publisher*
New Delhi | London | Philadelphia | Panama

Jaypee Brothers Medical Publishers (P) Ltd.

Headquarters

Jaypee Brothers Medical Publishers (P) Ltd.
4838/24, Ansari Road, Daryaganj
New Delhi 110 002, India
Phone: +91-11-43574357
Fax: +91-11-43574314
E-mail: jaypee@jaypeebrothers.com

Overseas Offices

J.P. Medical Ltd.
83, Victoria Street, London
SW1H 0HW (UK)
Phone: +44 20 3170 8910
Fax: +44 (0) 20 3008 6180
E-mail: info@jpmedpub.com

Jaypee-Highlights Medical Publishers Inc.
City of Knowledge, Bld. 237, Clayton
Panama City, Panama
Phone: +1 507-301-0496
Fax: +1 507-301-0499
E-mail: cservice@jphmedical.com

Jaypee Medical Inc.
The Bourse
111, South Independence Mall East
Suite 835, Philadelphia, PA 19106, USA
Phone: +1 267-519-9789
E-mail: jpmed.us@gmail.com

Jaypee Brothers Medical Publishers (P) Ltd.
17/1-B, Babar Road, Block-B, Shaymali
Mohammadpur, Dhaka-1207
Bangladesh
Mobile: +08801912003485
E-mail: jaypeedhaka@gmail.com

Jaypee Brothers Medical Publishers (P) Ltd.
Bhotahity, Kathmandu, Nepal
Phone: +977-9741283608
E-mail: kathmandu@jaypeebrothers.com

Website: www.jaypeebrothers.com
Website: www.jaypeedigital.com

© 2016, Jaypee Brothers Medical Publishers

Inquiries for bulk sales may be solicited at: jaypee@jaypeebrothers.com

Urology Instrumentation: A Comprehensive Guide

First Edition : **2016**

ISBN: 978-93-5152-181-5

Printed at Sanat Printers

Contributors

Abhishek B Ladhha MS DNB
Consultant Urologist
GBH American Hospital
Udaipur, Rajasthan, India

Abhishek G Singh MS MCh DNB
Consultant Urologist
Muljibhai Patel Urological Hospital
Nadiad, Gujarat, India

Amit S Bhattu MS DNB
Fellow in Endourology and
Laparo-robotic Urology
Consultant Urologist
Muljibhai Patel
Urological Hospital
Nadiad, Gujarat, India

Arvind P Ganpule MS DNB MNAMS
Vice-Chairman
Department of Urology
Muljibhai Patel
Urological Hospital
Nadiad, Gujarat, India

Jigish B Vyas MS DNB
Consultant Urologist and
Transplant Surgeon
Zydus Hospital
Sterling Hospital
Pramukhswami Medical College and
Shree Krishna Hospital
Nadiad, Gujarat, India

Jitendra V Jagtap MS DNB
Fellow in Endourology and
Laparo-robotic Urology
Consultant Urologist
Global Hospital,
Mumbai, Maharashtra, India

Mahesh R Desai MS FRCS
Medical Director and Managing Trustee
Muljibhai Patel Urological Hospital
Past President
Urological Society of India (USI)
Past President, Endourology Society Inc
Past President, Societe Internationale de
Urologie (SIU)
Nadiad, Gujarat, India

Raghuram Ganesamoni MS MRCS MCh
Fellow in Endourology and Laparo-robotic
Urology
Consultant Urologist
Ganesamoni Hospital
Nagercoil, Tamil Nadu, India

Rahul A Chrimade MS MCh
Consultant Urologist
Department of Urology
RR Hospital,
Nashik, Maharashtra, India

Ravindra B Sabnis MS MCh
Chairman
Department of Urology
Muljibhai Patel Urological Hospital
Nadiad, Gujarat, India

Shashikant K Mishra MS DNB
Fellow in Endourology and
Laparo-robotic Urology
Consultant Urologist
Chief, Uro-oncology Services
Muljibhai Patel Urological Hospital
Nadiad, Gujarat, India

Sujata K Patwardhan MS MCh
Professor and Head
Department of Urology
Seth GS Medical College and
KEM Hospital
Mumbai, Maharashtra, India

Forewords

Like all surgical subspecialties, the practice of urology encompasses a wide array of specific instrumentation. However, unlike many surgical disciplines, urologists perform unique endoscopic, robotic and open surgical techniques which require a myriad of basic instruments as well as complex endoscopes and single use instrumentation.

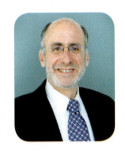

The text is a must for students as well as junior urologists as an ideal source to get full information on instruments in one location. In other words, this comprehensive guide is an ideal source to acquire all you required. Previously, it has been difficult to find a compendium of all the instrumentations specific to urology. Fortunately, the authors have answered this dilemma with a comprehensive text on urologic instrumentation including standard and advanced endoscopes, disposable instruments as well as devices specific for robotic surgery. Also included a thorough description of energy sources and sterilization methods, which are routinely used in urologic surgery both in the operating room and outpatient situations. Congratulations to the authors for compiling such an exhaustive review of urologic instrumentation.

Glenn M Preminger MD
Duke University Medical Center
Durham, North Carolina, USA

Improvements in urological instrumentations and accessories are occurring continuously due to the excellent collaboration between the physicians and our industrial colleagues. There is a pressing need for the residents and practicing urologists to both appreciate the improvements being made and how all these newer and improved devices fit into current clinical practice. This publication that you are holding right now meets this need and allows the urologists to have access to a

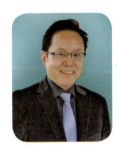

complete range of current instrumentations and accessories used in urology. Understanding the indication, optimal usage and complications associated with each device allows the urologists to improve his or her practice resulting in even better patient outcome posturological surgery.

Michael YC Wong
Associate Editor, BJUI Knowledge
Deputy Director, Asian School of Urology, Singapore

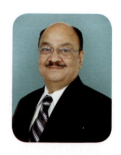

Necessity is the mother of invention. This adage is true for medical science.

Medicine is an ever-changing branch and concepts keep changing in a short period of time. This is particularly true for urology as a specialty. These thoughts are pertinent to the conception and execution of such a project. Such a book is the need of the hour for students intending to study urology as residents and appear for the MCh and DNB examination.

These students prior to appearing for the examinations currently have to scan through atlas, catalogues and number of books pertaining to instrumentation prior to taking-up examination. The book would benefit these students. In addition, the book would also be beneficial to young urologists intending to start practice and are undecided regarding the final choice of instrument.

The write-up of the book is such that the examination-going students would find it to be a source of information and answers for prospective questions during examinations. I am sure that the book would be an informative read. I congratulate the editors—Ravindra B Sabnis, Sujata K Patwardhan, Arvind P Ganpule, and of course all the contributors for this outstanding work.

Mahesh R Desai MS FRCS
Medical Director and Managing Trustee
Muljibhai Patel Urological Hospital, Nadiad, Gujarat, India

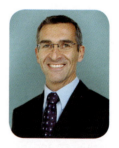

Urology has pioneered and contributed to many technological advances in surgery including surgical instrumentation and techniques such as endoscopy, laparoscopy and most recently, robotic surgery. These new technologies have radically changed surgical management and the minimally invasive approach has become increasingly utilized. Endourological and minimally invasive approaches now play an essential role and are the standard of care for the surgical treatment of certain pathologies such as kidney stones and prostate cancer, respectively. A large variety of instruments has been developed and is available, however, it is crucial for surgeons to master the use of these instruments in order to perform safe and effective surgery. The book including numerous educational illustrations, provides these essential surgical principles to urologists in training.

Olivier Traxer MD
Professor of Urology
Steeve Doizi MD
Assistant Professor of Urology
University of Paris VI (Pierre and Marie Curie University), Paris, France

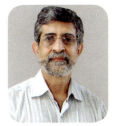

In over three and a half decades of urological practice, arguably my most satisfying and rewarding role has been that of teacher and guide to our trainees. Teaching is something one does out of passion and never as a duty or chore. I have known that the editor(s) of the book for many years and found them to be passionate and involved as a teacher. It is a pleasure for me to write the foreword on Urology Instrumentation.

Winston Churchill once said, "Give us the tools and we will do the job". As urological surgeons, our professional lives center around the tools we employ. As is true for any craftsman (and craftsmen we are in addition to our roles as care providers and scientists), familiarity and mastery over the use of tools, we use is an essential part of our competence. Although instruments per se, do not form a large part of the qualifying examination, a candidate's familiarity and confidence in handling the instruments, he/she is expected to use routinely, sets him/her apart as well trained.

I am sure that trainees will find a wealth of information in the book, which will help them in their examinations and practice.

Percy Jal Chibber
President, Urological Society of India (USI)
Head of Urological Services, Jaslok Hospital, Mumbai, Maharashtra, India

---

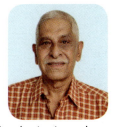

Ravindra B Sabnis, Sujata K Patwardhan and Arvind P Ganpule will have to be complimented for bringing out *Urology Instrumentation: A Comprehensive Guide*. The need for such a book has been felt over a long period of time. Though primarily intended for the trainees in urology, where knowledge of understanding of the various instruments is crucial, the book in its format can be hailed as God sent for all in urology at all levels.

There has been a recent avalanche as regards newer technologies in urology that involves many newer instruments made available. Proper handling of these instruments with an insight as to the nuances of the instruments that are being used are a necessity for all involved in using them. Such knowledge will help in keeping them in working order over a longer period of time, so essential for many developing financially strapped countries. The book gives it all. The armamentariums in urology from the past to the present have been addressed succinctly. Additionally, the usual pitfalls involved in usage of these instruments have been highlighted. There are 14 well-written chapters addressing specifically to one aspect that make reading not only pleasant but more meaningful. We have always read regarding instruments and their usage in bits and pieces taken from various sources. The book has given us the opportunity to understand all about the various instruments, we use at one stop.

I must once again admire the editors for the arduous task undertaken in bringing out the book. I am sure the book will be available on the desks of all urologists for frequent references and also become akin to a bible as far as trainees are concerned. Master your instruments and they will serve you better.

P Venugopal
Professor Emeritus (Urology) Kasturba Medical College (KMC)
Mangaluru, Karnataka, India

Preface

During various National Boards, University and mock examinations as an examiner, we realized that most students become shaky when they appear for instrument viva. This is probably because there is no dedicated book for reading. They go through various atlas/catalogues provided by companies, that contains lots of unnecessary information, and hence, students are under pressure to face this viva.

Over the years, we realized that there is need to have a book on this topic. We decided to write a small booklet to give information about commonly asked instruments in examination. While writing the booklet, suggestions came from many colleagues about not restricting scope of the book only to those examination-going trainees but expand it to give full information about all urological instruments. We accepted suggestions and decided to have this compressive guide of all urological instruments. We also decided to add chapters such as disposables, laparoscopic/robotic instruments, energy sources, sterilization methods, etc. so as to give value to the book.

Urology is rapidly advancing branch and it is more so in urological instrumentations. Within short-time, new instruments come which makes whole armamentarium quite big. In our attempt to provide updated information, we have referred to various catalogues and textbooks, however, as medical facts keep changing, newer things keep adding, some information may be lacking or may be old, hence the book should be viewed keeping this in mind.

We feel, the book will not only be useful to the trainees of MCh or DNB courses but also to all urologists, who wish to remain updated with various instruments in urology. We also feel that the book will be useful abroad especially in countries, where examination pattern is somewhat similar to ours.

It would be unfair, if we fail to acknowledge the hardwork of our assistant editors and contributors towards completion of the project. We thank Glenn M Preminger, Michael YC Wong, Mahesh R Desai, Olivier Traxer, Steeve Doizi, Percy Jal Chibber and P Venugopal for going through the book and writing forewords. We also thank M/s Jaypee Brothers Medical Publishers (P) Ltd, New Delhi, India to have accepted to publish this rather unusual book.

Ravindra B Sabnis
Sujata K Patwardhan
Arvind P Ganpule

Contents

CHAPTER
1

The Cystoscope and Accessories

INTRODUCTION AND BRIEF HISTORY

Maximilian Carl Nitze is credited with the invention of modern cystoscope, which was primarily used for inspection of the bladder. This was publicly demonstrated in 1879. It used an electrically heated platinum wire for illumination, a cooling system which used flowing ice water and telescopic lens for visualization. In 1887, following the invention of the light bulb by Thomas Edison, Nitze constructed a cystoscope that did not require the cooling system.

Cystoscopes are manufactured by various companies namely, Karl Storz, GmbH, Richard Wolf GmbH and Olympus Inc. We shall be describing the instruments by Karl Storz GmbH with some technical detailing from other manufacturers where ever necessary.

For many years, Karl Storz™ cystoscopes were utilizing the older nomenclature for sizes of the cystoscopes. In the nineties, the numbering of cystoscope sheath changed. Although the nomenclature changed, the actual size did not (Table 1). For the purpose of uniformity we will describe the new Storz numbering schema.

TABLE 1 The old and new schema for Karl Storz cystoscopes sheaths

Old schema	15.5	17	19	21	23.5
New schema	17	19	20	22	25
Color code	Yellow	Green	Red	Blue	White
Catheter capacities	1 × 5 Fr	2 × 5 Fr or 1 × 6 Fr	2 × 6 Fr 1 × 7 Fr	2 × 7 Fr 1 × 10 Fr	2 × 8 Fr 1 × 12 Fr

The parts of a rigid cystoscope assembly (Figure 1) are as follows:
1. Cystoscope sheath
2. Cystoscope obturator
3. Bridge
4. Light cable
5. Telescope

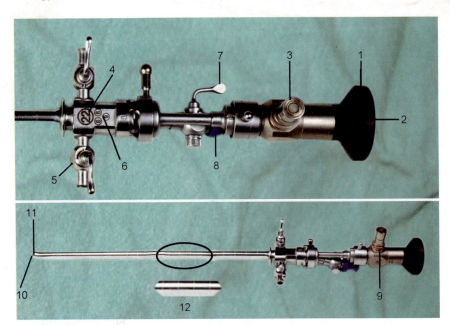

1. Ocular funnel
2. Ocular window
3. Light pillar
4. Number denoting the sheath size
5. Irrigation inlet and outlet
6. Number denoting the size of ureteric catheter that can be passed through the sheet
7. Stop cock of working channel
8. Working channel
9. Color code disk
10. Objective window
11. Beak
12. Marking on the sheath (1 cm apart)

Figure 1: Parts of a cystoscope

All cystoscopes are made of stainless steel alloy. The cystoscope sheath is calibrated in French (Fr), this is considered to be the outer circumference of the instrument in millimeters (mm). Fr is same as Charriere (Ch). This method of calibration was described by Joseph Frederic Benoit Charriere. Fr takes into consideration the diameter of the instrument.

One mm is equal to three French. It is also written as F, Fr or Ch.

THE CYSTOSCOPE SHEATH

The cystoscope sheath (Figure 2) will be discussed under the following headings:
1. Cystoscope sheath.
2. Beak.
3. Inlet and outlet vent.
4. Color code disk.
5. Numbering on the sheath and Albarrans sheath lever.

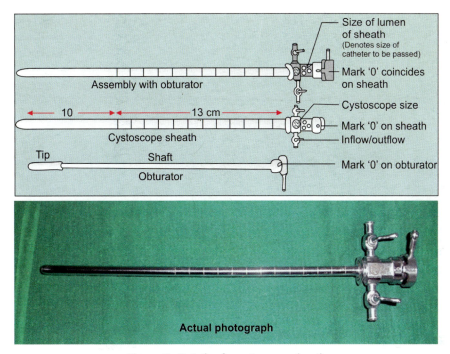

Figure 2: Details of a cystoscope sheath

1. *Cystoscope sheath*: The details of cystoscope sheath (Karl Storz, GmbH) are as follows:
   a. Length of an adult cystoscope sheath regardless of size is 22 cm. The cross section of the sheath is not round but oval. However, the size of the sheath is referred to in French(Fr), this can be considered as a 'misnomer' as mentioned, because if it is to be referred in French it should be circular contrary to its oval shape (Figure 2).
   b. *Markings on the shaft (Figure 2)*: The proximal 10 centimeters from the vesical end devoid of any markings. Markings are engraved on the sheath at every 1 cm thereafter for the next 13 cm. The markings help in estimation of prostatic urethral length (In comparison, VIU sheath has similar markings all along the length of the sheath).
   c. *Method to measure prostatic urethral length*: The cystoscope is introduced along the entire length. The cystoscope is withdrawn under endoscopic vision till the bladder neck. The marking on the external meatus is noted (Point A). Thereafter, the cystoscope sheath is withdrawn till the verumontanum and a note of the marking is done (Point B). The number of markings on the sheath between point A and point B is noted, this is the length of the prostatic urethra.

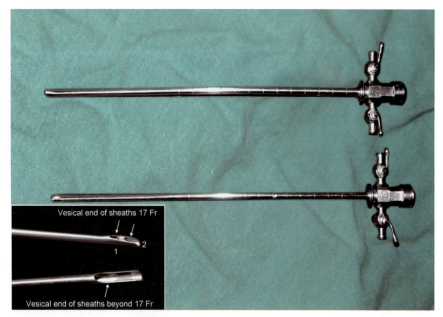

Figure 3: Types of cystoscope beak

  d. The distal end of the sheath is bulbous dorsally and smooth without sharp edge. This helps in atraumatic introduction of the scope (Figure 3). Such a design of the tip is essential if a instrument is to be passed under vision (without a obturator), e.g. cystoscope sheath, ureterorenoscope.

  If the beak is not of such design then that instrument should be passed through the meatus with obturator, e.g. VIU sheath, resectoscope sheath.

Salient features to remember regarding cystoscope sheath:

• Old and new nomenclature is changed without change in size
• All adult sheaths have same length
• Only 17 Fr sheath has different beak configuration, rest have same configuration.
• Bridges and telescopes remain same irrespective/regardless of size of sheath.

2. *Cystoscope beak*: Sheaths with size 19 Fr onwards are long oblique beaks, 17 Fr sheath is short beak sheath, this is used for female cystourethroscopy. The short beak is 2 cm in length (diamond shaped opening for irrigation at the beak with) while the long beak has a length of 2.5 cm. The gradual withdrawal of the cystoscope sheath helps in visualization of the urethra in females.

Longer beaks would result in leakage of irrigation fluid after introduction into a short female urethra leading to nondistension of the urethra and poor vision, this problem can be circumvented with shorter 17 Fr sheath (known as female cystoscope sheaths), this problem can also be circumvented by use of (Figure 4) the Nickel adapter used for female urethroscopy.

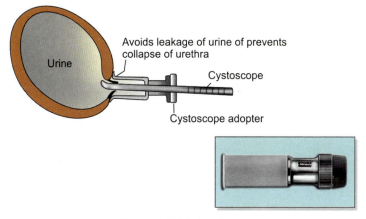

Avoids leakage of urine of prevents
collapse of urethra

Urine

Cystoscope

Cystoscope adopter

Figure 4: Nickel's adapter

The adapter should be pressed against the urethral orifice after insertion of the cystoscope to avoid leakage of irrigation fluid and the resultant collapse of the urethra.

3. *Inlet and outlet vent*: One for the inlet and one for the outlet allows ingress and egress of the irrigation flow which the surgeon can control (Figure 1).

4. *Color code disk*: This is a metal disk on which there is plastic color code cover. With prolonged use or repeated autoclaving it tends to get damaged.

5. Numbering on the sheath and Albarrans sheath lever:
   - Size of the sheath is indicated by a number written on the sheath at the level of inlet/outlet channel.
   - The numbers written in two circles behind the above indicate the largest size of the catheter, two of which can be passed simultaneously through the sheath.
   - Behind the above is a single circle with a numerical value, denoting the single largest catheter, which can be passed through the sheath.
   - The above catheter size are the maximum size with scope and Albarrans lever *in situ*, so if simple bridge is used maximal permissible catheter size will increase by 1 Fr. So the maximum size of catheter that can be passed through 19 Fr sheath with simple bridge is 7 Fr, (for 20 Fr is 8 Fr, for 22 Fr is 11 Fr and for 25 Fr is 13 Fr).
   - *Albarrans lever (Figure 5)*: It is Bridge with a deflecting lever, which can be used to deflect the ureteric catheter to align the catheter with the ureteric orifice. It has two channels through which two catheters can be passed simultaneously. A circular knob near the eyepiece end of the device is used to deflect the lever and thus, the ureteric catheter to up to 90°. Pointer on the knob tells the degree of deflection. Albarrans lever can be attached to sheath size 19 Fr or more.

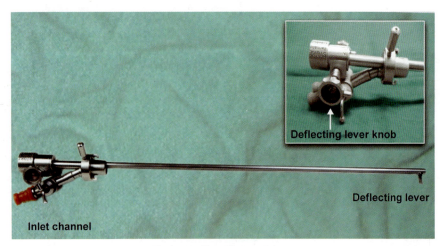

Figure 5: The Albarran's lever

  – *Locking knob on the sheath*: It has a zero (0) mark engraved which corresponds with same (0) mark on the obturator or the bridge (Figure 2).

Bridges (Figure 6)

Adult cystoscope bridges are universal and can fit into all sizes of sheaths. Length of bridge is 6 cm. Specially designed cystoscopes are available wherein the bridge and the telescope cannot be detached, they are called as 'integrated cystoscopes'. These cystoscopes have advantages of having a smaller shaft size with a comparatively larger working channel.

The advantages of detachable bridge are:

1. It helps in empting the bladder efficaciously.
2. It helps in passing larger size catheter after detaching the bridge.
3. It helps in attaching the Elick's evacuator for evacuation of stone fragments/clots/chips, etc.

Types of Bridges (Classification)

1. Without side channel
2. With one side channel
3. With two side channel.

Parts of Bridge

- *Telescope channel*: It accommodates the telescope.
- *Accessories' channel*: It is meant to pass the accessories such as ureteric catheter, wires forceps, etc. It has a rubber shod which help in easy passage of the instrument.

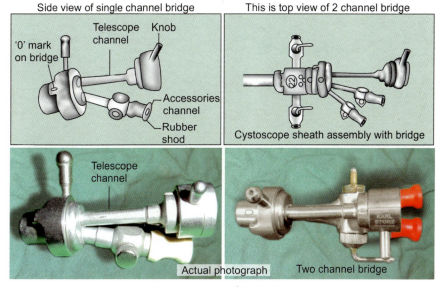

Figure 6: Parts of the bridge

OBTURATORS (FIGURE 7)

They are specific for a given sheath. Once attached to the sheath it makes the tip of the sheath smooth thereby snuggly fitting to it. The length of the obturator is 26 cm.

Parts of obturator are as follows:

- *Vesical end knob*: This helps in smooth atraumatic insertion of the cystoscope.
- *Shaft*: Connects the vesical end knob and the locking mechanism.
- *Locking mechanism*: Zero (0) should correspond to zero (0) of the sheath when locked.

Specifications of Obturators (Figure 7)

The obturator of 17 Fr sheath (new) has a smaller distal end without any groove. In addition, the sheath of 17 Fr sheath has a diamond shaped opening at the distal end which helps in irrigation egress. The obturator of 19 Fr sheath (new) onwards has a groove which helps in egress of irrigation. The sheath size is engraved on the obturator. The 17 Fr obturator has a smaller knob but is same in length. Rest of the obturators have same shape and length but vary in the size according to the size of the sheath. Points which differentiate a cystoscope, Sachse's and resectoscope obturator are detailed in Figure 7. The differentiation is based on size of the knob and the presence and absence of groove (Table 2).

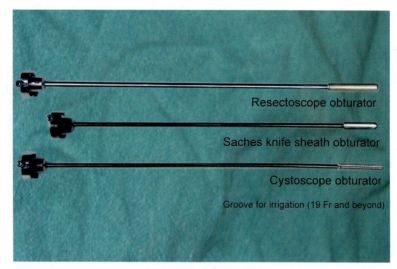

Figure 7: Types of obturator

TABLE 2 Difference in the type of obturators			
	Cystoscopic sheath obturator	*VIU sheath obturator*	*TURP sheath obturator*
Knob	Conforming to the beak of sheath	Rounded	Rounded
Groove	Groove for irrigation is present (19 Fr and beyond). 17 Fr sheath has no groove	Absent	Absent
Length	Equal to the sheath	Projects just beyond the sheath	Projects just beyond the sheath

SPECIAL TYPES OF CYSTOURETHROSCOPES AND ITS USES

Extended length cystoscope-urethroscope: The working length is 29 cm. It is 22 Fr, the color code is blue. The compatible telescope bridge has one instrument channel; it is for use of 10 Fr instruments. A catheter deflecting mechanism is also compatible with the extended length cystoscope-urethroscope, it is for use of 9 Fr instruments.

- *Continuous flow laser cystoscope-21 Fr (URO-LAS)*: The round tip configuration of the sheath and an 8 Fr working channel helps for easy urethral manipulation and insertion of laser with its accessories. The laser telescope bridge after Fraudorfer is compatible with the cystoscope.

THE TELESCOPES

The telescopes are classified depending on the viewing angle. They are available as 0°, 30°, 70°, 120° and 12° (Figure 8). Adult telescopes can be used with any adult sheaths. They need to be used with a bridge. The color coding for the telescopes are as follows, green code for 0°, red code for 30°, yellow code for 70° and white code for 120° for Storz (Figure 8). Even though the color codes seem confusing it is paramount for universal recognition. Straight forward telescopes (0°) is focused to view straight ahead, is usually used for urethroscopy. Forward oblique telescopes (30°) best affords visualization of the base and anterolateral aspect of the bladder, this is the most commonly used telescope. Lateral telescope (70°) to view the bladder dome.

It views structures around bladder neck like postprostatic pouch. Retrospective telescopes (120°) help to visualize the anterior bladder neck from inside. With conventional system, the viewing angle was relevant but with Hopkins 2, the use of 70° and 120° has gone down. In addition, with the use of flexible cystoscopes on the rise the 70° and 120° telescopes have become obsolete. These color codes differ with the make (Figure 8). The eyepiece can be fitted with a camera. The eye-piece is black in color and has the catalog number engraved on it. The light cable can be attached to the telescope directly. Size of telescopes available – 4 mm, 30 cm (fits in all cystoscope sheaths and VIU sheaths, resectoscope sheaths).

0°	Green
12°	Black
30°	Red
70°	Yellow
120°	White

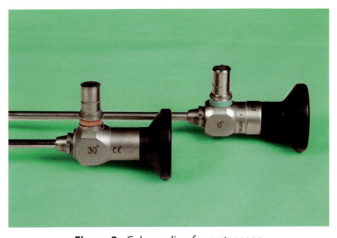

Figure 8: Color coding for cystoscope

The Rod-lens System (Figure 9)

In 1966, the collaboration between Karl Storz and Professor HH Hopkins led to the new design of rod-lens system. This was a major development for the progress of endourology since the description of cystoscope by Maximilian Nitze.

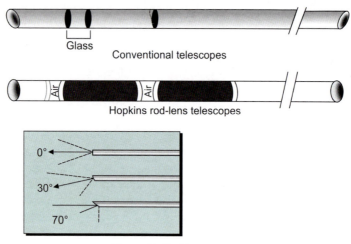

Figure 9: Rod-lens system

The key difference in the conventional optical system and the rod-lens system is that the Hopkins rod-lens system employs special glass rods with customized finished ends. The rod-lens system reduced the air spaces between lens with long rods of glass which were ground, contoured, and polished at both ends, there are short gaps of air in between. Once this endoscopic image is transported back through the telescope, it is magnified at the ocular lens. The degree of magnification is to some extent dependent on the diameter of the viewing lens.

The image and optical image transmission differs in rigid and flexible endoscopes. In the flexible endoscopes, typically there are two sets of fiberoptic glass bundles which are either coherent or noncoherent. The coherent bundles help in transmission of images, as a result the image of a fiberoptic scope has a 'honeycomb' appearance. This is called as the 'Moire effect'. The noncoherent bundles help in transmission of light.

Difference between Conventional and Hopkins Rod-lens System[1] (Table 3)

The Hopkins rod-lens system offers the following advantages over the conventional system:
1. Better light transmission offers images of improved quality and contrast.
2. Wide viewing angle offers better visualization of the structures.

TABLE 3 Comparison of conventional versus Hopkins rod-lens system

Conventional	Hopkins rod-lens system
Glass rods act as lens	Rod-lens, air space acts as lens
Thicker shaft profile	Smaller shaft profile
Narrow viewing angle	Wide viewing angle
Poor image resolution	Better image resolution

3. The image resolution is better.
4. Improvement in refractive index.
5. Increase in viewing angle.
6. Decrease in profile of telescope shaft.

Advantages of Hopkins II Lens

1. Wider viewing angles.
2. Lens diameter has been increased and air spaces have been decreased.
3. 30° Hopkins II covers areas which could be only seen by a 70° lens earlier.
4. Autoclavable.
5. Greater brightness.
6. Greater brilliance.
7. Higher resolution.

Basic structure of telescope (Figure 10).

Rod-lens are glued with special adhesive cement which is a special alloy, effectively making it water proof. The special adhesive helps in preventing permeation of water into the rod-lens system.

• *Light pillar*: Figure 11 shows the adapters and light pillars for various manufacturers. The light cable configuration differs with the make. Hence, the structure of light pillar varies. The use of adapters helps the use inter-changeable for example a specific custom made Wolf adapter can be used with the adapter on a Storz instrument.

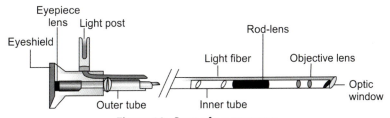

Figure 10: Parts of a cystoscope

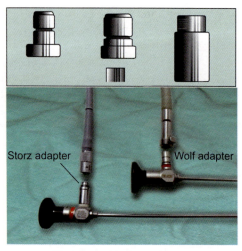

Figure 11: Various adapters

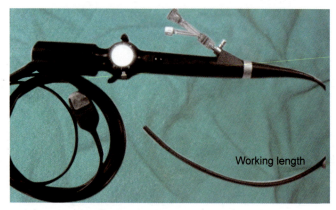

Figure 12: Flexible cystourethroscope

Parts of Telescope

- *Shaft*: Angulation at the tip varies depending on the viewing angle (diagram).
- *Eyepiece*: It is typically black in color, the size is universal and adapts to any camera head.

Flexible Cystourethroscope (Figure 12)

The advantage of flexible instrumentation is ease in patient positioning resulting in better patient comfort. It is useful in manipulation across difficult curves and high bladder necks and median lobes. The ability to flex the endoscope helps in complete visualization of the bladder easily. Within the shaft of a flexible cystourethroscope are generally three fiberoptic bundles—two noncoherent bundles of fibers that transmit light and a single coherent bundle of glass fibers that constitutes the imaging bundle. Unlike its rigid counterpart, the image obtained by the fiberoptic bundle is not a single image, but rather a composite matrix of each fiber within the bundle. The image obtained is analogous to a newspaper photograph—that is, it is composed of multiple dots merging into a single reconstructed image known as 'honeycomb' effect.[2] It is same as flexible nephroscope hence also called as flexible cystonephroscope. All are digital, they do not need a separate camera or light cable attachment. Specifications (Storz, Gmbh).

- Outer diameter—15.5 Fr
- Instrument channel—7 Fr

Direction of view 0°

- Field of visioin—110
- Working length—35–40 cm

The distal tip moves up for 180° and down for 140°.

The accessories which are compatible with flexible cystoscope are. All have to be flexible in nature:

- Grasping forceps—5 Fr, 73 cm
- Biopsy forceps—5 Fr, 73 cm
- Stone basket—5 Fr, 60 cm
- Ball electrode—4 Fr, 73 cm.

The flexible cystourethroscope can be sterilized with gas sterilization.[1,3]

Types

Logic (up is up). This means when the lever is turned down the deflection occurs downward and Antilogic (down is up). This means when the lever is tuned down the deflection goes up.

The cystoscope accessories are discussed in the chapter on accessories.

REFERENCES

1. Karl Storz catalogue, endourology, 5th edition, 1/97.
2. Babyan RK, Wang DS chapter one basic principles optics of flexible and rigid endoscopes Smith endourology, 2nd edition, Page 3.
3. Karl Storz catalogue, 5th edition, 1/97 Cyst 1B.

Visual Internal Urethrotomy, Otis Urethrotome and Meatotomy Instruments

SACHSE'S OPTICAL URETHROTOMY (FIGURE 1)

The Sachse's optical urethrotome assembly includes the outer sheath, obturator, zero degree telescope and a working element.
The details are as follows:

1. *Sheath*: The size of the Sachse's optical urethrotome sheath is 21 Fr (1 Fr or Chr is equal to 0.33 mm). This refers to the outer circumference of the metal sheath. The length of the sheath is 20 cm. In contrast to the cystoscope sheath the Sachse's sheath has markings throughout the length (20 markings) each

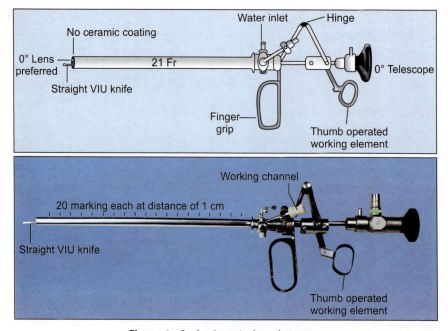

Figure 1: Sachse's optical urethrotome

at a distance of 1 cm. The sheath has a side working channel (top left side for right handed). The channel admits instruments up to 5 Fr. Cross section of the tip of the sheath is straight (not oblique or bulbous). A left handed surgeon can order a customized sheath (top right side instrument channel).

2. *Obturator*: The obturator of a Sachse's urethrotome is required while negotiating the meatus as the tip of the sheath is straight, thus a sheath introduced without obturator would be traumatic. The obturator in place smoothens the tip and helps in easy introduction of the urethrotome through the external urethral meatus. Once this is done obturator can be replaced by working element with lens *in situ*.

3. *Working element*: The thumb operated working element is used as this helps in maintaining the knife inside the sheath at rest and avoids injury to the urethra. The working element is same as used for transurethral resection of the prostate (TURP).

Blades (Figure 2)

The blades are usually double stem. They cannot be used with high frequency current

The types of blades are:

1. *Sachses' cold knife straight*: This is the most commonly used knife used for short segment bulbar stricture.
2. *Cold knife hook-shaped*
3. *Cold knife round shaped (half moon)*: It is useful for cases with bladder neck stenosis. Half moon knife because of its design cannot be passed under vision. It needs to be deployed when the Sachse's urethrotome is in place in the urethra. It cuts to and fro (while going in and coming out).
4. *Ludwik's straight knife waveform (Serrated)*: It is useful for dense strictures or core through urethrotomy.

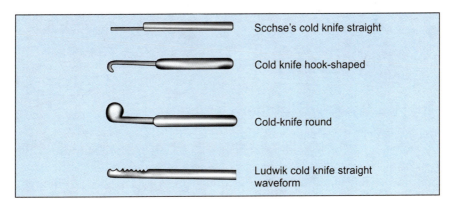

Scchse's cold knife straight

Cold knife hook-shaped

Cold-knife round

Ludwik cold knife straight waveform

Figure 2: Different types of VIU blades

Inlet Channel

The Sachse's optical urethrotome sheath does not have a outlet channel, it only has a inlet channel.

Accessories for a Sachse's Urethrotomy Sheath

1. *Half sheath (Figure 3)*: It is to be attached over the sheath. It increases the circumference and should be deployed in position prior to insertion. The size of this assembly becomes 23 Fr. After removal of the sheath it accommodates 16 Fr or less Foley catheter. It is used when one anticipates a difficult introduction of Foley's catheter.
2. *Continuous irrigation sheath*: It is a outer sheath to VIU sheath, similar to TURP outer sheath. It has multiple hole akin to a resectoscope sheath and a outlet channel for egress of irrigating fluid. It is useful in difficult urethrotomies when bleeding occurs and vision gets hampered, because in VIU sheath there is no outlet to irrigative fluid and also fluid is not able to enter the bladder due to tight stricture.

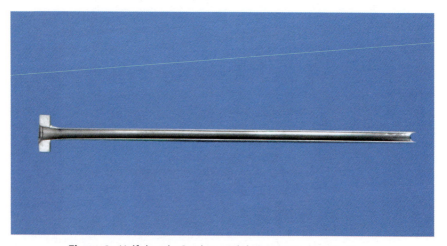

Figure 3: Half sheath: Can be used during optical urethrotomy

Otis Maurmyers Urethrotome[1] (Figure 4)

The instrument is commonly used to incise a narrow urethra. It is also used for managing urethral stenosis in females. The knife is inserted through the hub of the urethrotome and incises only tough tissues. The knife does not protrude beyond the surface of the instrument in a fully deployed position. The prerequisite for use of this instrument is the presence of a full bladder to avoid inadvertent incision of the bladder. The knife should be inserted with thumb pressing on the shaft of the knife as the knife enters the groove as shown in the figure.

The parts of a otis urethrotome are:

1. *Shaft:* The shaft is 16 cm in length and houses a hub/groove for passage of knife. The tip of the shaft is smooth, this avoids injury to the bladder. The shaft on the dorsal aspect houses a hinged calibrating device which maximally can dilate the urethra to 15–45 Fr. This is connected to the calibrating gauge on the external end. The knob at the tip of the instrument helps in passage of a filiform bougie. Size of the shaft is 14 Fr on rotating end, the knob at external end helps the shaft to open up. Once open maximum size achieved is 45 Fr. The minimal diameter of the urethra should be at least 16 Fr to admit this instrument. The bulbous tip gets detached and there is a threaded area which can be connected to filiform dilators and followers (Figure 4).

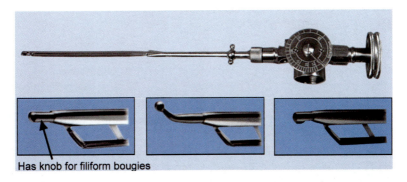

Has knob for filiform bougies

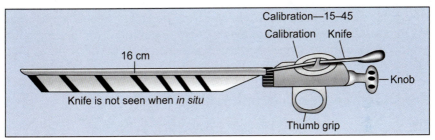

Figure 4: Otis urethrotome

2. *The external end:* The external end has a calibration gauge, a rotating knob, thumb grip and a knife hub. The maximum dilatation and incision that can be achieved is 45 Fr.

Knife has to be slided through the V shaped guider located over disk. Knife has to go into the groove.

REFERENCE

1. http://www.elmed.ro/upload/products/pdf/product_1319.pdf   accessed   on 28/08/2013.

TURP
Instruments

INTRODUCTION AND HISTORY OF TURP INSTRUMENTS

In 1909, Hugh Hampton Young developed a cold-cut punch for prostate resection, which was used blindly. Electrical cautery that could work underwater was first demonstrated by Edwin Beer in 1909. The second invention was amalgamated with the first in 1911, but the diathermy and resulting hemostasis was of poor quality, which limited its usefulness. It was Maximilian Stern who designed and named the first instrument as resectoscope. It had a tungsten wire. The idea of foot switch was first putforth by Davis. In 1932, Joseph F. McCarthy introduced the first modern resectoscope. His landmark contribution to innovation of the resectoscope was development of Bakelite sheath. Iglesias who happened to be Mccarthy student developed continuous irrigating resectoscope. Further, Captain George Baumrucker designed a spring mechanism for the working element with an action that was the reverse of the Iglesias mechanism (Resectoscope).[1]

Resectoscope Sheath (Monopolar)

The resectoscopes are available from a variety of manufacturers. The available sheath sizes are 22, 24, 26,28 Fr.

Parts of Resectoscope

Different ways of Classifying Resectoscopes

1. Depending on size 24 Fr, 26 (yellow) Fr, 27 Fr, 28 Fr (black)
2. Depending on beak (short or long or oblique)
3. Depending on sheath material (Teflon or MTC)
4. Depending on type of irrigation (Conventional or continuous).

1. *Depending on size*: Standard resectoscope sizes available are 24, 26, 27, 28 Fr. The 24 and 26 Fr are color coded yellow and used same loop which are also color coded yellow. The 27 and 28 Fr are color coded black and look the same loop which is colored brown. Now a 22 Fr integrated resectoscope is also available for small size urethra and its color coded white.

2. *Depending on types of beaks*
   - *Long beak:* These are similar to cystoscope beak but have no bulbous end. The long beak supposedly occludes the bleeders during resection. However, this design of the beak led to poor vision and is not commonly used.
   - *Short beak:* Optimization of the length was done to prevent the mentioned drawback of the long beak. This design has gone out of fashion.
   - *Oblique beak:* It has a short oblique end. Most modern resectoscopes have this design.

Vesical end of the resectoscope (Figure 1).

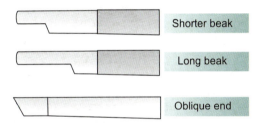

Figure 1: Various shapes of vesical end of resectoscopes

3. *Depending on materials of sheath*: During transurethral resection if the loop is still active (foot pedal pressed) and if it comes in contact with the sheath, it can damage and erode the sheath because of very high temperature. In addition it can transmit the current through the sheath if the insulation is breached or the sheath is conductive. Previously sheaths were made up of Bakelite, this material was fragile and hence susceptible to easy breakage. Then came Teflon which had better durability and was non- conductive of electricity. Later, metal sheath was tried, it gave good strength to the sheath but since metal sheath would conduct electricity it resulted in current leakage. In addition metal made the sheet heavy.

   Modern resectoscopes sheaths are made of MTC (Metal, ceramic and teflon). The distal portion is made of teflon which is nonconductor, rest of the sheath is metal, which gives strength, the inner portion of beak is coated with ceramic which is heat resistant and nonconductor.

4. *Depending on type of irrigation*: Depending on irrigation system mechanism they are classified as:

Conventional Irrigation

Does not have a outer sheath resulting in requirement for frequent emptying of the bladder.

Continuous Irrigation (Figure 2)

Outer sheath is added for drainage of irrigation fluid. First described by Iglesias in 1975. It enables resection to be undertaken as a continuous, uninterrupted process. It can be used as a conventional resectoscope after removing the outer sheath. Works on the principle of 2 concentric sheaths so that the irrigation

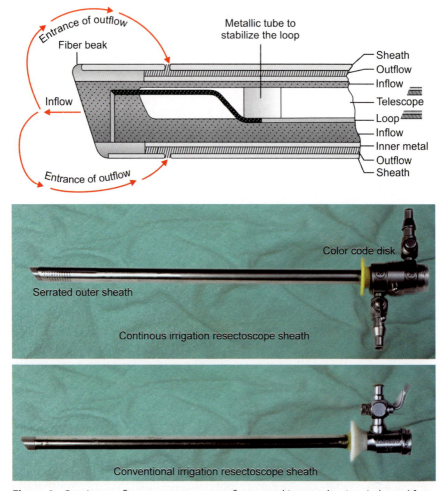

Figure 2: Continuous flow resectoscope top figure working mechanism (adapted from Blandys textbook of operative urology) and the bottom figure: actual photograph of the resectoscope

channel passes down the central sheath over the telescope and active electrode. The return flow enters the outer sheath just proximal to the beak of the instrument; the flow then passes between the 2 concentrically arranged sheaths to the exit tap. The advantages include the following. It avoids any build up of pressure inside the bladder, keeps field clear, quickens the procedure of transurethral resection and it will maintain the volume of bladder at a constant capacity for resecting bladder tumors (Figure 2).

What is a Rotating Resectoscope?

It is a resectoscopes that enables the urologist to rotate the working element and telescope to the desired position independently of the sheath. The result is no rotating components in the urethra and no entangled tubings due to rotation. This makes the procedure simpler.

Parts of Resectoscope Sheath

The resectoscope sheath generally consists of a cylindrical metal tube, the internal (vesical) end, which is protected from the current by a ring of insulating material. The vesical end is available in varying contours ranging from long beak to minimal obliquity. The insulating coating helps in preventing burns. A metal sheath may be responsible for burns to the urethral mucosa.

The types of insulated coatings are:
- *Bakelite:* The sheath for the original Stern McCarthy instrument was made of insulated material.
- *Teflon:* In Teflon sheaths small leakages can give rise to large leak of current.
- *Ceramic:* This material is currently used as a insulation coating.

External End of the Resectoscope (Figure 3)

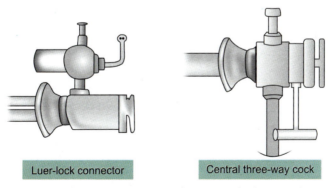

Luer-lock connector   Central three-way cock

Figure 3: External end of the resectoscope (Without central valve or with central valve)

Obturator (Figure 4)

It closes and smoothens the vesical end of the sheath and helps in instrumentation. This snugly fits into the sheath and helps in atraumatic insertion of the instrument.

They are of three types:

1. *Viewing obturator (SCHMIEDT):* It helps in introduction of sheath under direct vision, thus avoiding trauma to the urethra due to instrumentation and irrigation.

2. *Straight distending obturator (Leusch obturator):* Locking the obturator causes the rubber cuff to distend distal to edge of the sheath thus, covering its sharp edges, this reliably protects the urethra from trauma, by eliminating the 'little step' seen because of the gap between the sheath and the obturator, which avoids trauma due to the alignment because of the rubber.

3. *Hinged obturator (Timberlake):* Helpful for blind insertion of instruments, particularly in obstructing median lobe. When pressed obturator becomes angulated thus allowing negotiation at bulbar urethra and bladder neck.

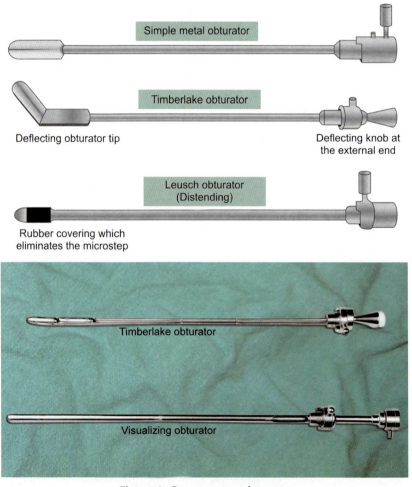

Figure 4: Resectoscope obturator

Working Element

Loop Control Mechanism

Three different types of loop control mechanisms are described. They are classified as passive or active or either as thumb operated or finger operated. The individual description is as follows:

1. *Rack and pinion system (Figure 5):* This was the original loop described by McCarthy. It works by to and fro movement of the lever. The loop requires a longer practice to master the art of resection. Not commonly in use.
2. *Thumb operated (Nesbit system)(passive)(Figure 6):* In this loop control mechanism, the Spring retracts the loop into the sheath, thus for cutting a tissue it requires the loop to be extended out of the sheath by pressure against the spring, the loop thereafter retracts on its own. This implies that cutting of the tissue is by passive retraction of the spring and hence the term 'passive'. In a resting state the loop is inside the sheath.
3. *Finger operated (Baumrucker system) (active)(Figures 7A and B):* In this loop control mechanism, the spring extends the loop out of sheath, the cutting is achieved by the manual retraction of the loop into the sheath. The cutting of tissue is by active retraction of the working element by the surgeon and hence the term 'active'. At resting state the loop remains outside the sheath. The preference of the loop to be used is a matter of surgeon preference.

What are the Advantages and Disadvantages of Active and Passive Working Element?

Advantage of active element:
As the movement is active, the resection is supposedly fast.

Disadvantage of active element:
- As the loop remain outside the sheath in resting state, the surgeon should be careful while operating.
- Since the cutting is active if surgeon exerts more pressure resection can become deep.

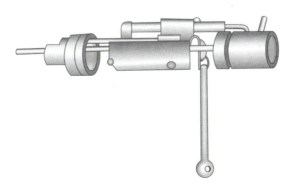

Figure 5: The rack and pinion working element

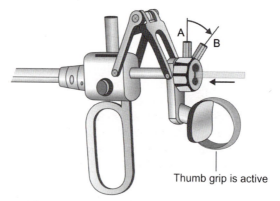

Thumb grip is active

Figure 6: Schematic diagram of thumb operated working element

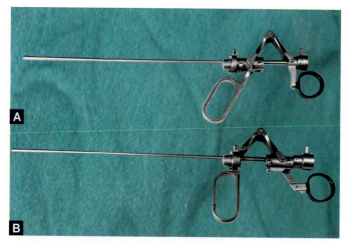

Figures 7A and B: (A) Finger operated working element; (B) Thumb operated working element

Advantages of Passive Element

- In resting position, the loop remains inside hence inadvertent damage to bladder is avoided if foot pedal is inadvertently pressed by the surgeon or the assistant.
- Since the cutting is passive the chips are cut in a controlled fashion.
- The same working element can be used for optical urethrotomy.

Disadvantage of Passive Element

Since cutting is passive speed of resection is slightly slower.

Cutting Loops

The loops are made of fine tungsten wire. The size is measured in mm. The size ranges from 0.35 mm (standard) and 0.30 mm (thin), 0.40 mm (thick).

Classification of Loops

1. Depending on size of sheath-24 Fr and 27 Fr.
2. Depending on color coding yellow is 24, brown-27.
3. Depending on size of wire-standard, thick and thin. The size of the loops are as follows 0.35 mm (standard) and 0.25 mm (thin), 0.40 (thick).
4. Depending on the telescope used (0° or 30°).

Most resection of prostate are done with 30° telescope, some bladder tumors at the dome are resected with 0° telescope. The loop for 0° is straight and 30° is curved.

All loops are color coded. 24 Fr and 26 Fr resectoscopes used yellow colored loops. 27 and 28 Fr resectoscope used brown color loop.

The path of passage of current is shown in Figure 8.

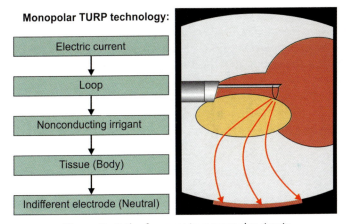

Figure 8: Path of current in monopolar circuit

The Broken Loop (Figures 9A to C)

If the loop breaks on passive arm-What happens?

- *If loop is broken at passive arm (Figure 9B)*: Current will continue to flow resection can be done, however loop will not be stable and will get angulated. Coagulation can be done without any problem.
- *If the loop is broken at middle of the curve (Figure 9C)*: The current will continue to flow, however resection cannot be done as only half part of loop is active.

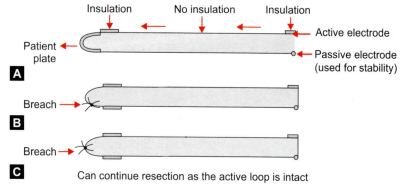

Figures 9A to C: Diagram showing what happens if a broken loop is used

What are uses of broken loop?
- It can be used if active arm is connected, for ureteric meatotomy.
- It can be used for BNI (Bladder neck incision).
- It can be used for posterior valve fulguration.

A few salient features for use include:
1. Thinner the loop, less the current required to cut, hence they are used when less charring is required. They are useful in resection of bladder tumor.
2. *Single stem or double stem*: Single or double stem do not make any difference in resection. In double stem the current only flows through active arms and passive arms gives stability.
3. Depending on sides of wire that standard, thick and thin.

Uses of Thin Loop

- When precise and sharp cut is required. Used for bladder tumor resection.
- Resection during TURP at the verumontanum (apical lobe resection).

Uses of Thick Loop

- Used for resection of bulk of adenoma.
- Eventually the thick loop becomes a thin loop after repeated use.

Types of Loops (Figure 10)

- *Standard cutting loop*: The standard loops are useful for transurethral resection of the prostate (TURP), whereas surgery to a prostatic adenoma demands the almost exclusive use of thicker loops so as to avoid change of loop during operation. Wear and tear occurs at the convex part of the loop and usually breaks in the center.
- *Collins Knife*: It used to incise bladder necks or TUIP. The incision is made in cutting mode thus achieving sharp linear cuts at the bladder neck.
- *Ball electrode (rolly ball/roller ball)*: This is used for achieving hemostasis after completion of the resection.

- *Conical electrode for point coagulation*: Helps in hemostasis.
- *Blunt curette*: This is for scraping off necrotic tissue.
- *Sharp curette*: This is for removing more firmly adherent slough and for drawing calculous debris into the sheath.
- *Mowing loop*: This is for resecting bladder tumors on the posterior wall.

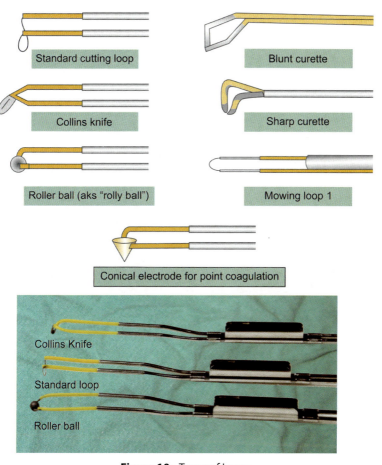

Figure 10: Types of Loops

Problems in Loop Angles

The loop electrode used for cutting should never be at more than a right angle to the insulated shoulders carrying the loop. The angle of the loop exactly corresponds to the angle of the beak, and the window of the telescope. The loop should retract less than 1mm inside the sheath so that it cannot approximate too closely to the telescope. The loop should retract inside the sheath to ensure that each cut of tissue is complete. If the loop is found to be at an obtuse angle to the insulated shoulder it will not retract inside the sheath and small tags of uncut tissue will remain.

High Frequency Cable

It gets attached on working element, the active arc of loop is longer and has insulation, right hole on high frequency cable accommodates the active long arm of loop. On left side there is no hole and the passive arm does not go inside and remain at the surface (Figure 11).

The active loop in adults is on the right side, 4 mm, 300 cm. In pediatrics, the active loop is on the left side (Surgeons view).

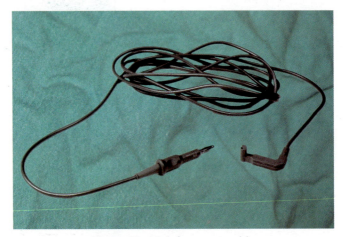

Figure 11: High frequency cable

Irrigating Fluids in TURP

Most commonly used fluids are glycine 1.5% in water (230 mOsm/L), sterile water. Other fluid which can be used are: 5% dextrose, mannitol, sorbitol, combination of mannitol and sorbitol.

Salient Features related to Absorption

- 20 mL/min absorbed.
- If 1 liter fluid absorbed then the drop in sodium level 5–8 mmol/L.
- A height of 60–100 cm above the patient is needed for irrigation and pressure of 2 kPa at the operative site is critical for fluid absorption.
- Not more 300 mL/min required for good vision–excessive irrigation pushed by the assistant avoided.
- Fluid absorption is proportional to the number of prostatic sinuses opened.
- Main driving force is hydrostatic force in operating area.

TURP SYNDROME

Definition

Sodium level after transurethral resection of the prostate (TURP) of < 125 mmol/L with two or more symptoms or signs of TURP syndrome (nausea, vomiting, bradycardia, hypotension, hypertension, chest pain, mental confusion, anxiety, paresthesia, and visual disturbance).

Risk reduction strategies to prevent TURP syndrome.

- Proper use of irrigating fluids
- Proper selection of patients
- Increased wariness in the part of anesthetist
- Newer modalities–bipolar TURP, laser TURP.

ACCESSORIES TO EVACUATE PROSTATE CHIPS

Ellik's Evacuator

Milo Ellik invented Elliks evacuator, he was resident under Alcock at university of Iowa. It consists of two glass bulbs connected to a rubber bulb and a connector for attachment to resectoscope sheath.

Method to use Elliks evacuator: It is to put in basin full of normal saline, rubber bulb is to be disconnected and filled with normal saline after creating negative suction, once this is done, it is reconnected to glass apparatus and placed under normal saline and a again filled by compressing the rubber bulb(creating suction). Once ready it is connected to resectoscope sheath and the rubber bulb is compressed and tip of the sheath is elevated in the bladder by depressing the shaft. The negative suction thus created sucks out all the prostatic chips and clots. It has to be filled completely with normal saline, if air enters evacuation does not take place properly (Figure 12A).

Modification of Ellik evacuator: It is commonly available. Normal saline is filled by pouring into the bottle after opening the cap, it has to be filled up to the brim of the connector. If air enters evacuation does not take place properly (Figure 12C).

Toomey syringe: They are glass syringes, have a metal catheter adapter. They are graduated with a 50cc capacity. The metal adapter fits on to the resectoscope sheath and it is used for evacuation of prostatic chips and clots by creating suction (Figure 12B).

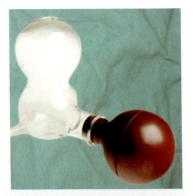

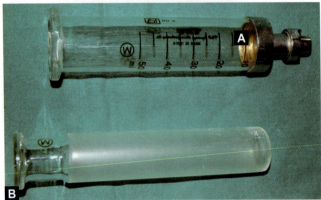

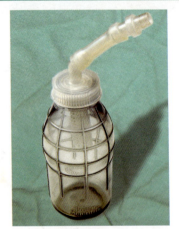

Figures 12A to C: (A) Elliks evacuator; (B) Toomey Syringe; (C) Modification of Elliks evacuator

REFERENCE

1. Blandy JP, Notley RG, Reynard JM. Blandy transurethral resection, 5th edition Chapter 1: History; 2005.pp.11-27.

Bipolar TURP

A bipolar electrode is defined as an electrode that has two active electrodes attached to a single support, and a structure that allows high-frequency electric current to pass through these two electrodes when electrified.

The bipolar technology uses the plasma arc for resection of tissue. The plasma is the fourth state of matter. It is a partially ionized gas containing *free electrons and cations*. The plasma is conductive. These gas molecules in plasma return to their initial state with emission of electromagnetic radiation of specific color which is orange for Sodium and blue or purple for Potassium.

The principles behind the resection in bipolar transurethral resection of the prostate (TURP) is as follows (Figure 1):

As the electrode is activated the current flows in the irrigation fluid as impedance is low in the saline. As the electrode is heated the air bubble forms around the electrode and whole electrode gets covered with air bubbles. Later current is conducted to air surrounding the electrode and then the plasma arc covers the electrode. Resection is done by the heat of plasma around the electrode.

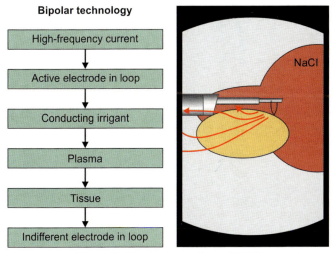

Bipolar technology

High-frequency current
↓
Active electrode in loop
↓
Conducting irrigant
↓
Plasma
↓
Tissue
↓
Indifferent electrode in loop

NaCl

Figure 1: Bipolar technology of TURP

IRRIGATION IN BIPOLAR TURP

As the irrigating solution used in bipolar TURP is normal saline there is no risk of TUR syndrome. However, it is to be remembered that this does not mean that there is no fluid absorption in bipolar TURP. So resection time has to be limited in patients who have co morbidities which may decompensate in fluid overload stage like congestive cardiac failure or renal failures.

ADVANTAGES OF BIPOLAR TURP

- Less conductive trauma so a lower rate of bladder neck stenosis or urethral strictures
- Elimination of TUR-syndrome
- Lower risk of capsular perforation has there is decreased stimulation of pelvic floor
- Better visual orientation by reduced coagulation depth
- Self-cleaning of the loop by high energy level at plasma ignition.

LIMITATIONS OF BIPOLAR TECHNOLOGY

- Higher risk of conductive trauma if current is deviated via sheath and insufficient lubrication.
- Risk of recurrent bleeding due to smaller coagulation zone.

There are different types of bipolar electrodes:

These differences are by the way in which the active and indifferent electrodes are arranged:

1. Two different loops (parallel or opposite)
2. Using the distal end of the resection loop
3. Using the working element of the resection shaft.

Types

Quasi-bipolar: The current does not flow exclusively between two electrodes (i.e. definition of bipolar electrosurgery). Instead the current runs to a negative pole through sheath of the resectoscope. e.g. olympus TURis system (Figure 2):

Olympus TURis System

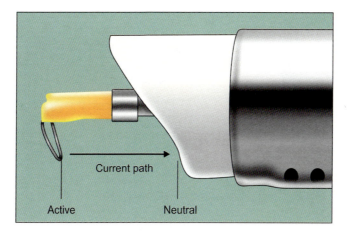

Figure 2: Olympus electrode

- *Plasma kinetic resection loop by Gyrus*: It uses a single platinum-iridium loop as active electrode, whereas on the same axis (axipolar) the distal end of the loop (stainless steel electrode separated by a ceramic insulator) serves as neutral electrode. This loop is designed for single use (Figure 3).

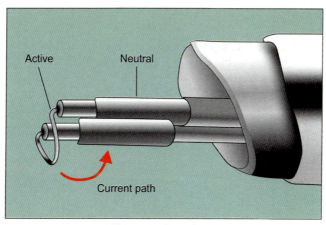

Figure 3: Gyrus loop

- *Karl Storz bipolar resectoscope loop*: It has 2 oppositely facing loops with passive electrode as counterpart. This loop is designed for multiple uses (Figure 4).

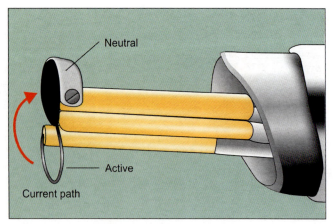

Figure 4: Karl Storz electrode

- *Bipolar button electrode* for transurethral vaporization of prostate (Figure 5)

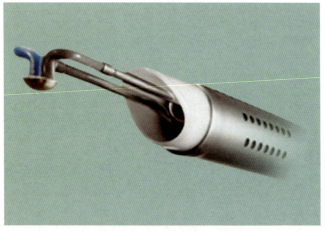

Figure 5: Button electrode

CHAPTER
5

Cystolithotrity Instruments

HISTORY AND BRIEF INTRODUCTION

Jean Civiale was a urologist practicing in France in the nineteenth century and is credited with invention of surgical instrument lithotrite and performed transurethral lithotripsy. This is considered to be the first minimally invasive surgery. The instrument which he developed contained three prongs to grasp a stone. The instrument was capable of making a number of holes in the stone.

Bladder stones can be managed either by urethral route, suprapubic route or by open approach. The suprapubic approach is preferred in multiple stones or large stone bulk. The transurethral route offers a plethora of options with regards to the energy source. The stone can either be crushed with stone crushing forceps or broken by ultrasound, pneumatic or laser energy lithotrite. In pediatric age group laser and pneumatic are preferred energy sources.

Nomenclature of Various Procedures

1. *Cystolitholapaxy*: Intact removal of stone.
2. *Cystolithotrity*: Mechanical crushing of the stone.
3. *Cystolithotripsy*: Breakage of stone with energy source.
4. *Cystolithotomy*: Open removal of stone.

Stone Crushing Forceps (Figure 1)

It is available as a single action jaw. The stone crushing forceps fits in 25 Fr cystoscope sheath. This forceps can be used for smaller stones and for crushing fragments after use of lithotrite. After removal of forceps evacuation is possible through the sheath with evacuator. The surgeon should not grasp stones larger than the size of the jaw, as it may damage the instrument. The assembly requires 30 degree telescope. It is less robust than Maurmyers stone punch. While crushing stones and it is important that bladder is not empty, stone is grasped, instrument is rotated to ensure that the mucosa is not caught in the jaws.

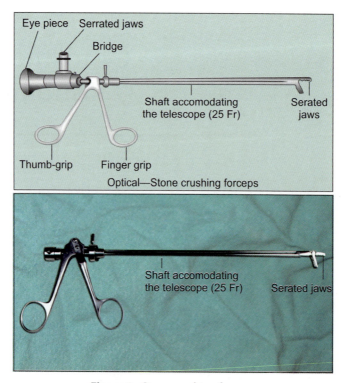

Figure 1: Stone crushing forceps

Hendrickson's Classical Lithotrite (Figure 2)

This instrument has to be passed blindly; it has to be used with 70 degree scope. It is Cumbersome to use. It is passed blindly like a dilator, hence there is a high chance of creating a false passage in urethra. If jaws get stuck it may even

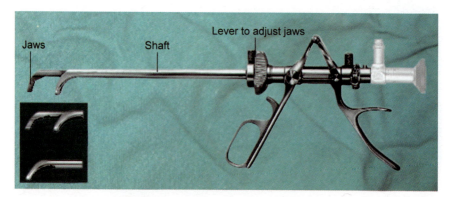

Figure 2: Hendrickson's classical lithotrite

need open surgical removal. This instrument is not used nowadays because of high rate of complications and availability of better instruments.

Maurmyers Stone Punch (Figure 3)

It is complete with its own sheath, working element and inserting obturator (with bridge). Hence becomes costly. It is sturdy therefore bigger stones can be crushed. Movement is forward, backward (vis-à vis-upward and downward movement in stone crushing). The instrument requires a zero degree telescope. The parts of the instrument include (Figures 3A and B):
1. A punch working element.
2. Punch sheath with central valve, 25 Fr straight beak with obturator.

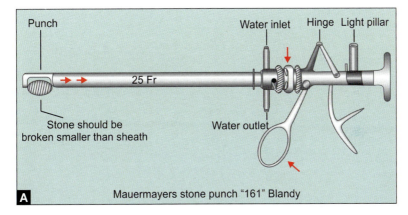

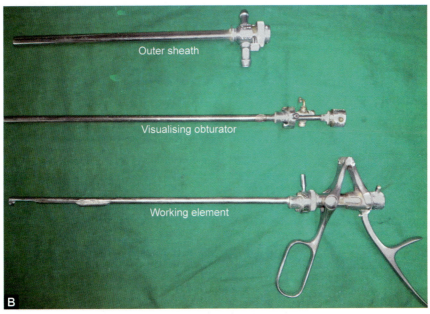

Figures 3A and B: Maurmyers stone punch

The stone can be broken so that it becomes small enough so that the stone can be pulled out through the punch sheath or can be washed with the evacuator. It requires to be introduced with visualizing obturator.

With the advent of lithoclast, nephroscope with lithoclast is used for management of bladder stones, making stone crushing devices less useful.

PCNL Instruments

INSTRUMENTS

The key instruments required for successful completion of a Percutaneous nephrolithotomy (PCNL) are:

1. Access needles
2. Tract dilators
3. Nephroscope (rigid and flexible)
4. Accessories, Guidewires, forceps, etc.

Access Needles (Figure 1)

The access needle helps in gaining optimal access and also offers space for passage of guidewire. Typically; the needle has two parts, a shaft and a stylet. Traditionally, they are classified as two parts and a three part needle (Figure 1). The needles can also be classified depending on the configuration of

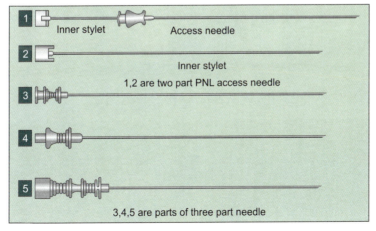

Figure 1: Access needles

the tip which can be either beveled or diamond tipped. In general, the shorter needles have better control. Longer needles are necessary for obese patients and in a situation where a ultrasound guided puncture is contemplated. The triangulation technique requires a longer tract and hence it requires a longer needle. The alternative access needle system uses a 21-gauge primary access needle; these needles are compatible with a 0.018 guidewire.

Types of Needles (Figure 2)

- *Initial Puncture Needle-3-Part Bevel Tip*: These are the first instruments used for gaining access. A 0.035" guidewire is used with it. Initial puncture needle is 18 gauge, it is 20 cm in length and has 3 part with a bevel tip. The bevel helps in ensuring entry of guidewire into the pelvicalyceal system (PCS). The beveled tip should be facing the crystals in the ultrasound for acoustic visualization of the needle. The disadvantage of using a beveled needle is that the needle tends to bend toward the bevel. In contrast, the diamond tipped needle does not deviate in either direction. This is not used nowadays as there is no specific advantage of three part needle over two part needle.

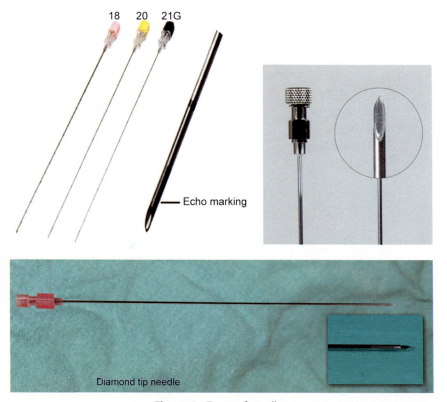

Figure 2: Types of needles

- **Initial Puncture Needle-2-Part Trocar Tip (Cook Urology 2010 Domestic product catalogue pg 125):** This is the most popular needle. The needle is 20 cm in length; it is 18 gauge, 2 part trocar tip. The color code is pink for 18 gauge, yellow for 20 and black for 21 (Figure 2).
- **Chiba Needle–Three part Bevel Tip[1]:** It has stylet, inner sheath and outer sheath. Outer sheath is of shorter length. It is used for fluoroscopy guided puncture. Puncture is made with 21 Gauge needle since it is longer in length. When perfect puncture is made as confirmed by efflux of urine on withdrawal of stylet. Then outer sheath is advanced over the inner sheath. Once it reaches PCS the stylet and inner sheath is taken out and the operator proceeds for dilatation. Advantage of 21G needle is that even when multiple attempts are made to obtain PCS access, it would theoretically cause less damage to kidney, less bleeding and less chance of AV fistula as compared to 18G needle. Though this has not been proven in any study. The needle was developed at the University of Chiba, Japan. This needle is also called as a skinny needle and is used for opacification of the PCS.

PCNL Tract Dilators

The dilators are used for creation of PCNL tract. The types of dilators to be used are dictated by the size of stone and the degree of hydronephrosis and size of tract you want to make. The type of dilator to be used is a matter of surgeon's preference.

The types of dilators to be used are:
- Fascial dilators
- Screw dilators
- Amplatz dilators
- Telescopic metal dilators (also known as Alken dilators)
- Balloon dilators.

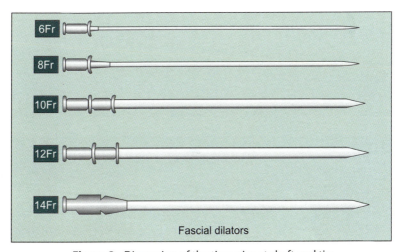

Fascial dilators

Figure 3: Dimension of the tip varies at shaft and tip

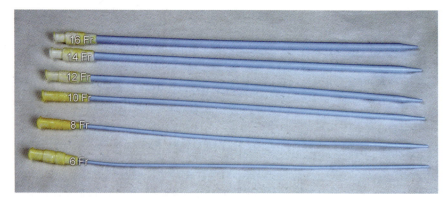

Figure 4: Fascial dilator

Tract Dilators

Fascial dilators (Figures 3 and 4)[2]
Available from 6 to 16 Fr polytetrafluoroethylene (PTFE), (Cook Medicals Inc, IN, USA) in size, they are useful for tract dilatation after puncture and placement of guidewire. Fascial dilators have an elongated conical tip and opening at the tip which accommodates the guidewire.

Once the access is achieved and guidewire is placed, the dilators are passed sequentially. The dilators are cheap but theoretically are associated with more bleeding, as each dilator is removed and replaced with one larger dilator until complete dilatation is achieved. As every time the dilator has to be removed and replaced the chance of bleeding due to loss of tamponade of the tract being dilated increases.

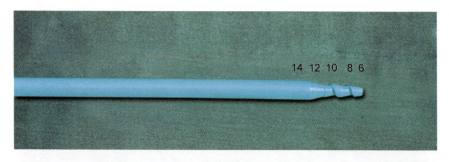

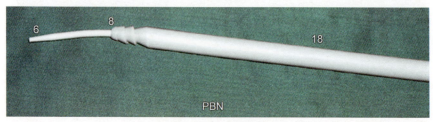

Figure 5: Screw dilators

- **Screw dilators (Figure 5)**[3]

They have a screw shaped tip. They are available in 3 sizes size 6 Fr to 12 Fr, 6 to 14 Fr and 6 to 16 Fr (6 implies the size of tip and 12 implies the size of the shaft). Even bigger dilators are available.

Amplatz Renal Dilator Set (Figure 6)

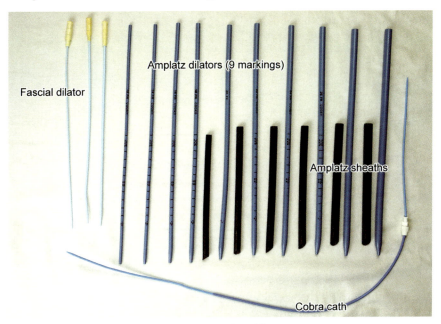

Figure 6: Amplatz dilator

They are used for progressive dilatation of nephrostomy tract prior to percutaneous kidney stone removal. They are radioopaque dilators and sheaths. They have a short tapered tip with smooth surface to reduce tissue trauma. A typical dilator set consists of an 8 Fr radioopaque tetrafluoroethylene (TFE) catheter (also known as cobra catheter), the dilators range from 12 Fr to 30 Fr, the Amplatz sheaths range for 24, 26, 28 and 30 Fr dilators. The sheaths are not numbered, however conventionally same size Amplatz sheath snugly fits over same size Amplatz dilator, e.g. 24 Fr Amplatz sheath will fit over 24 Fr Amplatz dilator. Radioopaque TFE catheter (Cobra catheter) acts as a guide for dilators 12F–30F, radioopaque TFE catheter (8 Fr) allows safety wire placement. They are 30 cm in length, however long Amplatz dilator with length of 32 and 40 cm are available (for obese patients). Smaller sheaths 14 to 20 Fr are now available. The length of sheath is 16 cm. The length of longer sheath is 20 and 30 cm (use for obese patients). Thus, once the puncture is made, guide wire is passed, tract dilated up to 10 Fr by using serial fascial dilators 6 Fr–8 Fr–10 Fr. Then cobra catheter (8 Fr) is passed in PCS. Over this catheter Amplatz dilators are passed sequentially one-by-one. Once the desired size dilatation is achieved by a dilator, over it corresponding Amplatz sheath is passed and dilator removed.

Metallic Serial Telescopic Dilators (Figures 7A and B)

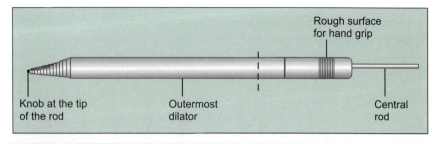

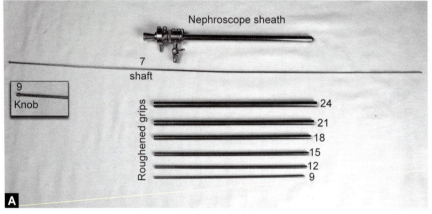

Figure 7A: Top: Schematic of Alken's dilators over Alken rod; Below: Alken's telescopic metal dilator

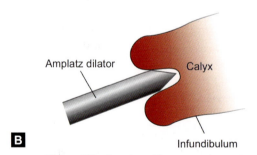

Figure 7B: Amplatz dilator entering calyx

The set consists of a central rod and serial metal dilators. The rod is 58 cm and can be either rigid or flexible. The most commonly used are the rigid rod which gives sturdiness required during dilatation. The entire unit resembles an assembled collapsed radioantenna after all the dilators are assembled. The dilators are advanced over a central rod which is 7 Fr in diameter and with a rounded knob which is 9 Fr in diameter. The central rod is placed over a stiff guidewire; the dilators are available in an increment of 3 Fr depending on the make (sarting from 9 Fr Upto 24 Fr). Additionally, 27 and 30 Fr size dilators can be ordered (Karl Storz, GmBh). After placement of guidewire, rod is passed with the advancing bulbar end. The first dilator being 9 Fr, it does not overshoot the knob of the central rod. The inner end of each dilator is designed in such a way that it does not go beyond the previous dilator and hence beyond the knob of the rod. Outer end of each dilator has serrations (holding grip) (approximately one inch) which allows optimal grip while dilating the tract. Each dilator is designed in such a way that they snugly fit over one another and do not traumatize the tissue during dilatation. Since the dilators snugly fit over each other and do not overshoot the knob of the rod, on withdrawing the rod all the dilators come out with the rod.

These dilators are cheap and allow complete dilatation upto calyx. The rigidity of this system offers it to be an effective dilator even in tough tissues such as in previously operated cases. The dilatation can be done upto the desired size and a sheath placed thereafter. Over the last dilator either a snugly fitting nephroscope sheath or an appropriately sized Amplatz sheath can be passed. Alternatively after removing all the dilators, Amplatz dilator and its sheath can be introduced over a rod.

The operator should be aware of the shortcomings of this system which include possibility of kinking the glidewire. In Amplatz system initial cobra catheter is passed. Over this catheter sequential, Amplatz dilatation is done upto desired size and then Amplatz sheath placed. While in Alken system a rod is passed over the guidewire and then serial dilatation done over which a nephroscope sheath is passed and PCNL is carried out. However, often dilatation is done by Alken system and over which Amplatz sheath is kept. If more force is applied then rod may advance further upto the medial wall of pelvis causing perforation. In the Amplatz system, the tip of the dilator is one inch conical and hence the tract is underdilated as the full shaft does not enter the PCS system. This assumes importance particularly if stone is occupying the whole calyx or narrow infundibulum. Every time the dilator is taken out there may be bleeding from the tract. This dilatation is time consuming.

Balloon Dilatators (Figure 8)[4]

These are radial dilators unlike other dilators which are axial dilators. The balloon dilators work by lateral compressive force rather than a lateral shearing force. After the initial puncture and placement of wire the tract has to be dilated up to 8 Fr with facial dilators and then balloon dilation catheter is introduced. High-pressure balloons are capable of developing pressures up to 15 to 30 atmospheres of pressure; the length varies up to 15 cm and diameters of 10 to 12 mm. With single balloon inflation, the entire access tract is dilated. They are placed over stiff guidewire. The distal end of balloon is placed close to collecting system (as close to stone bearing calyx as possible) and balloon is inflated by a luer lock controlled inflation device. Before introduction of catheter the Amplatz sheath should be back loaded from the renal end (it is not possible to pass the Amplatz sheath later). Finally Amplatz sheath is placed over the balloon and balloon is removed. The advantage of these dilators is

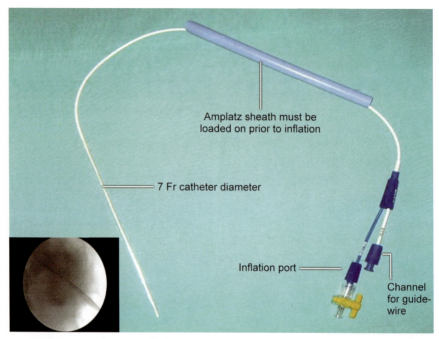

Figure 8: The parts of a ballon dilator inset shows the fluoroscopic view

that dilatation is rapidly achieved and they are easy to use. The disadvantage is that balloon has a tapered end, so dilatation upto entry calyx may not be complete, especially when enough length of glide wire is not parked in kidney. Balloon dilators tend to be less effective in dense retroperitoneal scarred tissue, in addition they are expensive.

Guidewires or glide wires: The guidewires are key accessories in preparation of any endourological procedure. The type of guidewire to be used depends on the access to be gained. The details have been mentioned in chapter on accessories.

Accessories for percutaneous nephrolithotomy: These would be discussed in chapter on accessories.

Nephroscopes

Varieties of rigid and flexible nephroscopes from different manufacturers are available. It is necessary to know the advantages and disadvantages of each to select a best instrument in a selected case.

The rigid nephroscopes have a rod lens system for imaging. The eye piece can be parallel to the nephroscope working channel or it can be oblique. The eyepiece of oblique variety is suitable for direct viewing as accessories can be inserted easily. The eyepiece of parallel variety is useful when endovision is used (this fact holds true when one is using a camera without a beam splitter). Oblique eye piece suits a beam splitter camera.

Types of Nephroscopes (Figure 9)

Classification

The nephroscopes can be classified as:
1. *Depending on the make*: Karl Storz, Richard Wolf, ACMI (Olympus)
2. Size of the nephroscope.

Major differences in Wolf and Storz nephroscopes are:

All wolf telescopes (of a nephroscope) are integrated with a sheath and hence can be used as an independent unit without the sheath over it. Storz

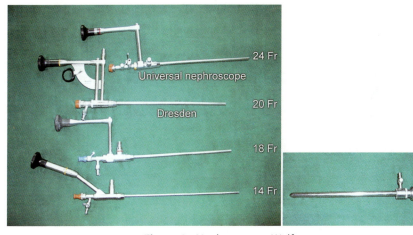

Figure 9: Nephroscopes: Wolf

nephroscopes have a sheath and the telescope and hence are not integrated, Storz recently has introduced a similar design of a slender nephroscope.

The parts of nephroscope are:
1. Sheath
2. Telescope.

Traditionally, the sizes of nephroscope mean the size of the sheath. Richard Wolf nephroscope models are called as universal nephroscope and are available in various sizes.

Adult Nephroscopes by Richard Wolf, GmBh, Tutllingen Germany.
1. Percutaneous low pressure universal nephroscope (Model Marberger):[5] It is 27 Fr in size and has a 25 degree down viewing telescope. It has an oval working channel through which 4 mm instrument can be used.
2. *Percutaneous universal nephroscope*:[6] The available size is 24 Fr sheath with channel accommodating 3.5 mm instrument. The viewing angle is 20 degree.

3. *Percutaneous universal nephroscope (Model Dresden):*[7] It has a 20.8 Fr sheath with larger working channel for instruments up to 3.5 mm. The working channel is oval in cross section. Angle of vision is 12 degree down (diagram of the grip). Although slender it has the same sturdiness as bigger nephroscope. The channel size is 3.5 mm and the design is ergonomically better because of the valve retainer.

4. Invisio® Smith Digital Percutaneous Nephroscope.[8]

This is a advanced scope, much lighter than traditional scope (470 gm verses 935 gm) effectively decreasing the fatigue during long procedure This also helps the surgeon to use nondominant hand-to-hold scope and use dominant hand to manipulate instruments.

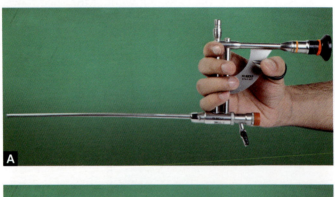

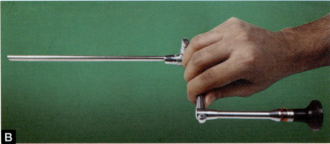

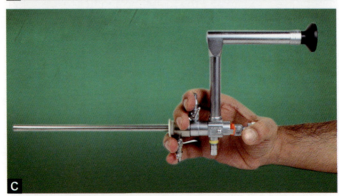

Figures 10A to C: Different grips of nephroscopes: (A) Wolf Dresden; (B) Wolf 24 Fr nephroscope; (C) Storz 24 Fr nephroscope

Difference in 24 Fr, 27 Fr and 20.8 Fr is 20.8 is to be held in a vertical manner) (Figures 10A to C)

The terminology "continuous irrigation" irrigation nephroscopes.

All nephroscope if used with sheath become continuous. The sheaths have side holes at the distal tip which allows egress of irrigation through the outlet channel. The nephroscope with sheath can be used with Amplatz of size more than 24 Fr.

Nephroscopes by Storz[9] (Figure 10 C)

The angle of vision in all Storz nephroscope is six degree, regardless of size. The available sizes are 22, 24 and 26 Fr. The eyepiece can be either parallel or oblique to the axis of the nephroscope (length available: 19 cm or 24 cm or 25 cm). Unlike Wolf these nephroscope cannot be used without sheath, as they are not integrated hence the water from the irrigating channel comes out at the proximal end and also accessories from the spraight channel are not aligned with the distal end. In Storz nephroscopes the light pillar is directed to the floor and the inlet channel toward the ceiling.

Miniperc

Although there is no consensus regarding definition for Miniperc, tract size less than 20 Fr is considered miniperc. Storz miniperc nephroscope is conceptualized by Naegle whereas the Wolf is conceptualized by Lamhe.

Storz miniperc is also called as modular miniature nephroscope system (Figures 11 and 12) with automatic pressure control. It is available in three sizes 15/18 Fr and 16.5/19.5 Fr and 21/24 Fr sheaths are available (Figure 13). This describes inner and outer circumference of the sheath. It comes with its own dilators with end hole accommodating the guidewire. Each sheath has its own dilator which has got end hole accommodating guidewire. The other component of the assembly include telescope with 6.7 Fr working channel for instrument upto 5 Fr with 22 cm length. There is an irrigation channel on sheath as well as on the working channel. However, the telescope can be used with any appropriate size Amplatz sheath. Eye piece is oblique.

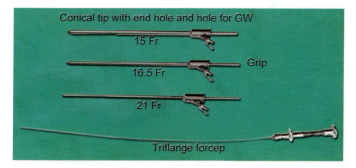

Figure 11: Storz miniperc sheath with dilator

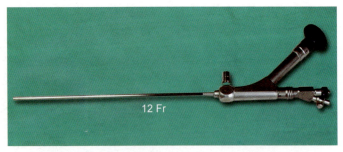

Figure 12: Storz miniperc dilator with Amplatz sheath

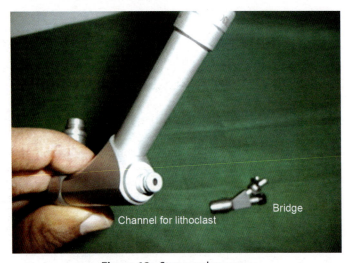

Figure 13: Storz nephroscope

Wolf minipercs nephroscopes are available in two sizes. Outer sheath size of 15 and 18 Fr (Figures 14 and 15). It comes with its own dilators with end hole accommodating the glide wire. Nephroscope is common with 12 degree angle and 6 Fr working channel and 14 Fr in size. However, the telescope can be used with any appropriate size Amplatz sheath. Very useful for stones in renal pelvis and staghorn calculi, can be used in children and adults, made up of titanium and stainless steel to decrease the weight of instrument. It has offset eyepiece.[10]

Accessories of Miniperc (Storz and Wolf)[11] Figures 16A and B

2 mm and 5 mm diameter forceps are available (alligator type or triflange type or mouse tooth type).
Because of small size of forceps these are very delicate and liable to damage very easily. Stones can also be removed with baskets.

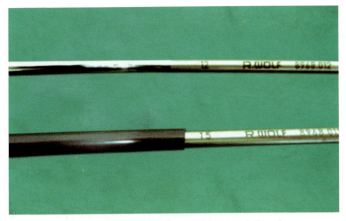

Figure 14: Wolf miniperc dilators and sheath

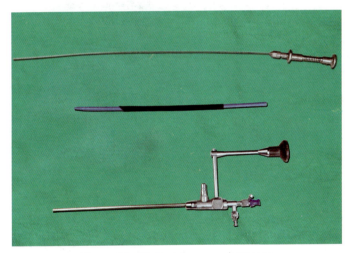

Figure 15: Wolf miniperc nephroscope

Microperc[12]

The parts of microperc assembly include:

- 3-part all-seeing needle, consisting of micro-optics 0.9 mm in diameter with a 120-degree angle of view and resolution up to 10,000 pixels (Figure 17).
- Needle, including the shaft, with outer diameter of 1.6 mm (4.85 Fr), slightly larger than the diameter of a standard 1.3 mm needle.
- The highly flexible fiber-optic telescope contains 10,000 fiber-optic bundles and can be bent over itself without causing damage (Figure 18).

There is an outlet from the connector to an irrigation pump (Figure 19).

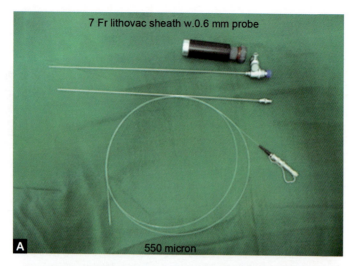

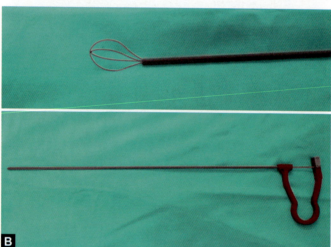

Figures 16A and B: Miniperc accessories

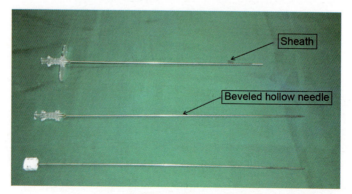

Figure 17: Three part needle

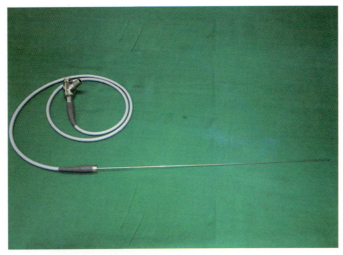

Figure 18: Fiberoptic telescope for microperc

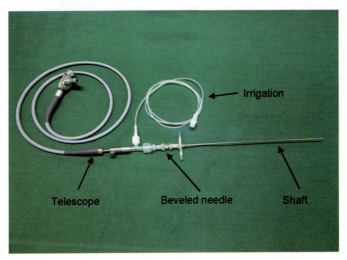

Figure 19: Microperc assembly

ULTRA MINI PCNL

It consists 3.5 Fr telescope which is mounted inside a 6 Fr sheath (LUT-GmbH, Germany). The inner telescope sheath has two side ports. One is used for irrigation and the other one for passing laser fiber. Telescope is connected to standard camera system. The outer sheath is 11 to 13 Fr sheath (Figures 20A to C).

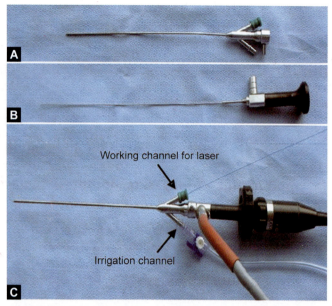

Figures 20A to C: Ultra Mini PCNL Assembly: (A) Inner sheath; (B) Telescope; (C) Inner sheath with telescope attached to camera light and irrigation

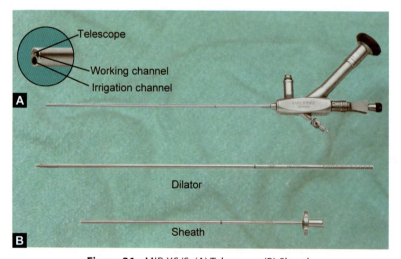

Figure 21: MIP XS/S: (A) Telescope; (B) Sheath

MIP (Minimally Invasive Percutaneous Nephrolithotomy) XS/S

Karl Storz™ 7.5 Fr nephroscope, 2 Fr working channel and 3 Fr irrigation channel. Uses fiber optic system and is 24 cm in length. It has Pre-fabricated dilator and sheath 8.5 Fr/9.5 Fr and 11/12 Fr (Figure 21).

REFERENCES

1. Cook Urology 2010 Domestic product catalogue pg 124.
2. Cook Urology 2010 Domestic product catalogue pg 50.
3. http://www.devoncath.com/Urology_dilatorssets.html accessed on 20/08/2013.
4. http://www.bostonscientific-international.com/templatedata/imports/collateral/Urology/oth_pcnl_01_ur_us.pdf accessed on 28 Aug 2013.
5. http://www.bostonscientific-international.com/templatedata/imports/collateral/Urology/oth_pcnl_01_ur_us.pdf accessed on 28 Aug 2013
6. Richard Wolf Catalogue pg.D740.305
7. Richard Wolf Catalogue pg.D740.303
8. http://www.gyrusacmi.com/user/display.cfm?display=product&pid=9849&catid=76&maincat = Video&catname = Percutaneous% 20Nephroscopes accessed on 28/08/2013.
9. Storz Urology product catalogue pg.150/151.
10. Richard Wolf Catalogue pg.D740.501).
11. Richard Wolf Catalogue pg.D780.901
12. J Urol. Single-step percutaneous nephrolithotomy Microperc: the initial clinical report 2011;186(1):140-5. Desai MR, Sharma R, Mishra S, et al.

FURTHER READING

1. Desai M. Ultrasonography guided punctures with and without puncture guide. J Endourol 2009;23:1641-3.
2. Desai MR, Sharma R, Mishra S, Sabnis RB, Stief C, Bader M. Single step percutaneous nephrolithotomy(Microperc): the initial clinical report. J Urol 2011;186(1):140-5.
3. Rassweiler J. Ipad assisted percutaneous access to the kidney using marker based navigation: Initial clinical experience. Eur Urol 2012;61:627-31.
4. Sountoulides PG, Kaufmann OG, Louie MK, et al. Endoscopy guided percutaneous nephrostolithotomy: Benefits of ureteroscopic access and therapy. J Endourol 2009;23(10):1649-54.
5. Olcott EW, Sommer FG, Nape S. Accuracy of detection and measurement of renal calculi: In vitro comparison of three dimensional spiral CT, radiography and nephrotomography. Radiology 1997;20:419-25.
6. Mishra S, Sabnis RB, Desai M. Staghorn morphometry: a new tool for clinical classification and prediction model for percutaneous nephrolithotomy monotherapy. J Endourol 2012;26(1):6-14.
7. Karami H, Rezaei A, Mohamaddahosseni M, et al. Ultrasonography guided percutaneous nephrolithotomy in the flank position verus fluoroscopy guided percutaneous nephrolithotomy in the prone position: A comparative study. J Endourol 2010;24(8):1357-61.
8. Agarwal M, Agrawal MS, Jaiiswal A, et al. Safety and efficacy of ultarsounography as an adjunct to fluoroscopy for renal access in percutaneous nephrolithotomy (PCNL) BJU international; 2011:108;1346-9.
9. Desai MR, Jasani A. Percutaneous nephrolithotripsy in ectopic kidneys. J Endourol 2000;14(3):289-92.

10. Xu Y, Wu Z, Yu J, et al. Doppler ultrasound guided percutaneous nephrolithomy with two step tract dilatation for management of complex renal stones Urology, 2012;79:1247-51.

11. Castaneda WR, Espenan GD. How to protect yourself and others from radiation In: Smith AD, Badlani G, Bagley D (Eds). Smiths Textbook of Endourology, 1st edition. Section 1 Chapter 3, St Louis: Quality Medical 1996:21-8.

12. Kahn F, Borin JF, Pearle MS, et al. Endoscopically guided percutaneous renal access:"Seeing is believing" J Endourol 2006;20(7):451-5.

13. Grasso M, Lang G, Taylor FC. Flexible ureteroscopically assisted percutaneous renal access. Tech Urol 1995;1:39-43.

14. Desai MR, Sharma R, Mishra S, et al. Single-step percutaneous nephrolithotomy (Microperc): the initial clinical report. J Urol 2011;186(1):140-5.

15. URL:Surgimedik medical systems http://www.surgimedik.com/ProductDetails. aspx?PID=86&CID=yYut//BrHa8=)

16. URL:Cook medical/ catalog page: http://www.cookmedical.com/uro/dataSheet. do?id=1941

17. URL: Cook medical: http://www.cookmedical.com/uro/dataSheet.do?id=1940

18. Falahatkar S, et al. One-shot versus metal telescopic dilation technique for tract creation in percutaneous nephrolithotomy: comparison of safety and efficacy. J Endourol 2009;23(4):615-8.

19. Aminsharifi A, Alavi, M, Ghasem Sadeghi, 1S Shakeri, and F Afsar, J of Endourol 25(6);2011:927-931.

20. URL:Cook medical systems:http://www.cookmedical.com/uro/familyListingAction. do?family=Wire+Guides).

21. Richard wolf medical systems URL: ww.richard-wolf.com/en/human-medicine/ urology.html

22. GYRUS ACMI Medical Systems URL:http://www.gyrusacmi.com/acmi/user/display. cfm?display=product&pid=9849&catid=76&maincat=Urology&catname=Percuta neous%20Nephroscopes.

Semirigid Ureteroscopy

INTRODUCTION

Hugh Hampton Young visualized upper urinary tract using a 9.5 Fr cystoscope in a male child with megaureter in 1912.[1] In 1979, Lyon et al used the first dedicated ureteroscope that was made by Richard Wolf Medical Instruments.[2] The original ureteroscopes used rod-lens system for image transmission. These instruments were larger in size and caused 'half-moon' effect while reaching the upper ureter. The later generations of ureteroscopes used flexible fiber optic bundles for both image (coherent) and light transmission (non-coherent). These ureteroscopes were smaller in caliber and did not distort the image even while bending. These ureteroscopes were called semirigid or mini-ureteroscopes. Dretler and Cho described the first semirigid ureteroscope or 'mini-scope' in 1989.[3]

EVOLUTION OF URETEROSCOPES

Goodman first reported rigid ureteroscopy in 1977 using a pediatric cystoscope.[4] The first endoscope specifically for ureteroscopy was designed by Richard Wolf Medical Instruments in 1979.[5] This instrument was 23 cm long and had 13 Fr sheath for inspection and 14.5/16 Fr sheath to allow insertion of instruments for stone removal. In 1980, Enrique Pérez Castro in collaboration with Karl Storz Endoscopy, developed a 39 cm ureteroscope which could reach renal pelvis.[6] Most of the initial ureteroscopes had interchangeable 0° and 70° telescopes. With the development of 8 Fr ultrasonic probes, these probes were used blindly to fragment stones after an initial inspection using ureteroscope. In order to allow small rigid probes through a straight channel in ureteroscope, telescopes with offset eyepiece were developed. The first ureteroscope with fiber optic imaging system was introduced by ACMI in 1985.[6] Once the rod-lens imaging system was replaced with fiber optic, the half-moon effect was eliminated. Later on, compact ureteroscopes, which integrated rod-lens telescope into the ureteroscope to reduce the outer diameter without compromising the size of working channel, were developed. Initially pneumatic and subsequently laser came into the picture. Once laser was developed, the need for a large working channel decreased and dual channel ureteroscopes with separate channels for flow and accessories were developed. Recent ureteroscopes have a high density of coherent fiberoptic bundles to improve vision and smaller outer diameter. All mordern ureteroscopes are semirigid and have optical fibers. Old rigid ureteroscopes had rod lens system which is now obsolete.

CLASSIFICATION

All semirigid URS have size described as 2 digits, e.g. 7/8.5 which means the tip is 7 Fr and shaft is 8.5 Fr. Every scope is small in size at tip and increases in size proximally. Each make has different way of transition of this size from tip to base. Common size of a URS are 6/7.5, 7/8.5, 8/9, 8 etc. Length of URS can be short or long. Short are generally 35 cm and used for females whereas long are generally 45 cm and are used for males.

Semirigid ureteroscopes can be classified based on size, make and channel.
1. According to make (Storz, Wolf, Olympus, Scholly)
2. Depending on channel
    Most ureteroscopes have a straight or oblique channel.
    Straight channel: Allows use of rigid pneumatic lithotripsy probes.
    Oblique channel: Also called as uretero-laser scopes.

Parts (Figure 1)

1. *Eyepiece*: Straight, oblique or lateral offset.
2. *Body*: It has a light post and working channels.
3. *Working channels*: Ureteroscopes have either a single larger channel or two separate channels. Dual channel also allows the simultaneous use of laser fiber and a basket.
4. *Sheath*: 7/8.5 Fr-Tip is 7 Fr (length varies) and shaft is 8.5 Fr-Wolf measures at the distal tip while Storz measures where the working channel ends (diagram).
5. Currently Wolf has three varieties of ureteroscope—needle (4.5/6 Fr), ultrathin (6/7.5 Fr) and dual-channel (6.5/8.5 Fr).

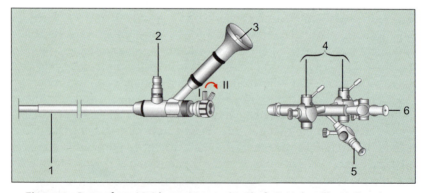

Figure 1: Parts of semirigid ureteroscope. 1. Shaft; 2. Light pillar; 3. Eyepiece; 4. Inlet + Outlet top; 5 and 6. Working channel

6. *Tip design*: General principles of tip of the instruments:
   Angulated tip: This helps to negotiate stricture and any meatus in atraumatic manner, e.g. Cystoscopes, Ureteroscopes. The angulated end is engaged initially and then the instrument is lifted up.

Karl Storz 7 Fr/9/9 Fr semi-rigid ureteroscope:

It is available in two lengths—34 and 43 cm. The distal end is angulated, rounded tip for smooth insertion into ureteric orifice. The telescope is of

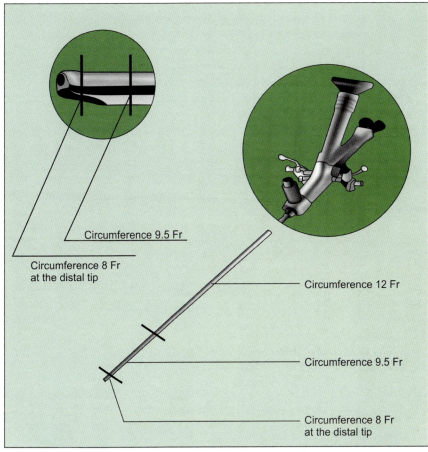

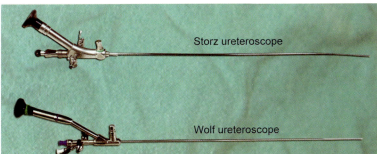

Figure 2: Specifications of Karl Storz endoscopes

fiberoptic system with a 6° angle of view at the tip. The tip measures 6.5 Fr without the working channel. The instrument sheath is 7 Fr in size for the distal 6 cm length, with an unobtrusive step to 9.9 Fr towards the proximal part. The sheath is conical in shape for strength and durability. The light post is just proximal to the proximal end of the sheath. There are two irrigation ports which open into the large working channel for maximum flow.

They are at right angles to the instrument to avoid cluttering of tubings and instruments. The irrigation port has an optional flow control stop cock for precise control of irrigation. The instrument ports are variable with quick release coupling and self-closing sealing system. The working channel is 4.8 Fr in size and allows rigid instruments up to 4 Fr. The eyepiece is offset to make instrument handling easier (Figure 2).

The other ureteroscopes currently available with Karl Storz are:
1. *8 Fr ureteroscope*: It has a 7 Fr distal tip. The instrument sheath is 8 Fr with a step to 12 Fr. Working channel is 5 Fr.
2. *9.5 Fr ureteroscope*: It has a 8 Fr distal tip. The instrument sheath is 9.5 Fr with a step to 12 Fr. Working channel is 6 Fr. Otherwise it is similar to the 7 Fr ureteroscope.
3. *9.5 Fr Michel ureteroscope*: It has a 9 Fr distal tip. The instrument sheath is 9.5 Fr with a single step to 12 Fr. It has a large central working channel with right-angled irrigation port and an additional separate 2.3 Fr irrigation port on the underside. The working channel allows simultaneous use of 2 and 3 Fr instruments or a single 6 Fr instrument.

Types of eyepieces

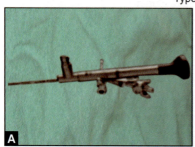

A

Direct view eyepiece

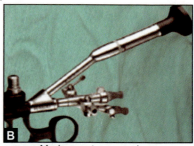

B

Marberger type eyepiece

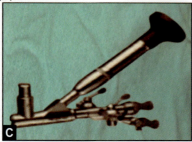

C

Bichler type eyepiece

Figures 3A to C: Types of eyepieces

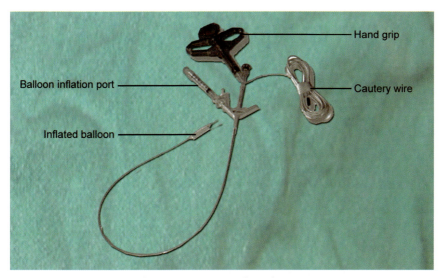

Hand grip

Balloon inflation port

Cautery wire

Inflated balloon

Figure 4: Acucise endopyelotomy

4. *7 Fr 'Laserscope'*: 8.4 to 9.9 Fr conical sheath with a 7 Fr tip diameter. It has a 2.4 Fr irrigation channel on left side. The 3.4 Fr working channel allows instruments up to 3 Fr. The eye-piece is straight. It is especially suitable for laser ureterolithotripsy (Figure 3A).

Richard Wolf ureteroscopes:

1. *6/7.5 Fr compact operating fiber uretero-renoscope*: This ureteroscope has a distal sheath tip of 6 Fr with atraumatic head shape and 5° angle of view and size increases to 7.5 Fr proximally. The sheath is stepless. There is a common oval shaped irrigation and working channel which allows a single instrument up to 4 Fr or two instruments of 2.4 Fr size.

   The eyepiece is either laterally offset (Marberger) (Figure 3B) lateral (Bichler) (Figure 3C) or direct view. There is an automatic valve for introducing instruments which avoids the need for opening and closing instrument port and leak of irrigation fluid during instrument exchanges. This instrument is available in two lengths—31.5 cm and 43 cm.

2. *8/9.8 Fr compact operating fiber uretero-renoscope*: This is similar to the previous scope except that the distal sheath tip is 8 Fr; angle of view is 12° and with oval irrigation and instrument channel allows one 5 Fr or 2 x 3 Fr auxiliary instruments. The eyepiece is either laterally offset (Marberger), lateral (Bichler) or direct view.

3. *8.5/11.5 Fr Marberger compact operating fiber uretero-renoscope*: In this instrument the distal sheath tip is 8.5 Fr, angle of view is 12° and with oval irrigation and instrument channel allows one 6 Fr or 2 x 4 Fr auxiliary instruments.

4. *6.5/8.5 Fr dual operating channel (DOC) ureteroscope*: This instrument is available with a straight or 45° lateral eyepiece and with 31.5 or 43 cm length. Its channel allows one 4 Fr or 2 x 2.4 Fr instruments.

5. *4.5/6.5 needle ureteroscope*: This ureteroscope has a tip design which is similar to other Wolf ureteroscopes. The tip is 4.5 Fr and shaft is 6 Fr. The viewing angle is 5° and insert capacity is 3 Fr. It is available with either parallel or 45° offset eyepiece and 31.5/43 cm lengths.

Olympus Ureteroscopes

The tip is atraumatic and sheath is stepless. The direction of view is 7°. The available sizes are 6.4/7.8 Fr shaft with 4.2 Fr channel and 8.6/9.8 Fr shaft with 6.4 Fr channel. These ureteroscopes are available with angles or straight eyepieces. The available lengths are 33 and 43 cm.

Accessories

These will be described in accessories chapter (cup biopsy forceps, spring forceps, alligator forceps, brush biopsy basket, bugbee, etc.).

Instruments used in Retrograde Endopyelotomy

Retrograde endopyelotomy can be performed using ureteroresectoscope, acucise device with holmium laser. Among these, holmium laser endopyelotomy is the most commonly used nowadays.

Ureteroresectoscope

The overall arrangement is similar to a routine resectoscope. This instrument can be used to incise strictures, resect ureteral tumors, or perform endopyelotomies or ureteral meatotomies. It has an 11.5 Fr sheath with irrigation channels, working element with attachments for cold knife or insulated electrocautery knife and a telescope. It was available in 27 cm and 43 cm working lengths. These instruments are not in use now and are no longer available.

Acucise Endopyelotomy (Figure 4)

Acucise device has a diameter of 6 Fr and length of 78 cm. The balloon is 10/24 Fr and cutting wire is 150 micron diameter and 3 cm in length. There is a side port for instillation of contrast. A radiofrequency cable is attached to the underside of the catheter. The balloon has radiopaque markers to properly align the balloon across pelvi-ureteric junction after contrast study. The wire is placed poster laterally and pure cutting current activated at 75 watts for incision and balloon left inflated for 2 minutes. Then an endopyelotomy stent is placed over guidewire. A tamponade catheter of 7 Fr in size and 78 cm long with a balloon of 13/30 Fr size and 4 cm length is supplied along with the device for tamponading bleeding.

REFERENCES

1. Young HH, McKay RW. Congenital valvular obstruction of the prostatic urethra. Surg Gynecol Obstet. 1929;48:509.
2. Lyon ES, Banno JJ, Schoenberg HW. Transurethral ureteroscopy in men using juvenile cystoscopy equipment. J Urol. 1979;122:152-3.
3. Dretler SP, Cho G. Semirigid ureteroscopy: a new genre. J Urol. 1989;141:1314-6.
4. Goodman TM. Ureteroscopy with paediatric cystoscope in adults. Urology. 1977;9:394.
5. Lyon ES, Banno JJ, Schoenberg HW. Transurethral ureteroscopy in men using juvenile cystoscopy equipment. J Urol. 1979;122:152-3.
6. Pérez-Castro Ellendt E, Martinez-Piñeiro JA. Transurethral ureteroscopy. A current urological procedure. Arch Esp Urol. 1980;33:445-60.

8

Flexible Ureteroscope

TYPES OF FLEXIBLE URETEROSCOPES

1. *Conventional*: It is a fiberoptic flexible ureteroscope. The light is carried to the tip by a set of noncoherent fiberoptic bundles and image is carried back by a set of coherent fiberoptic bundles.
2. *Digital*: The newer generation of flexible ureteroscopes have replaced the image carrying fiberoptic bundles with a camera sensor at the tip of the instrument. The image is thus carried as electronic signals. In these ureteroscopes, the camera is placed at the tip of the ureteroscope and the image is carried as electrical (digital) signal to the processing unit. Thus the coherent fiberoptic bundle is replaced by electric fibers. It is also called chip at the tip technology (Figures 1A to C).

Basic Design of a Flexible Fiberoptic Ureteroscope

Flexible ureteroscope consist of an elongated plastic-coated endoscope sheath containing optical components such as the objective lens and the image guide as well as the light-transmitting glass fibers. It also has one or two channels for insertion of instruments and irrigation of fluid.

Optical System

It is comprised of three different parts:
1. Objective lens.
2. Image guide, a precisely arranged glass fiber bundle for transmitting the image.
3. Ocular lens.

Parts of a Conventional Fiberoptic Flexible Ureteroscope

1. *Eye piece (ocular lens) and focusing component*: The eyepiece magnifies the virtual image and makes the image visible for the viewer. It allows for image focus adjustment.
2. *Hand piece*: Hand piece has the following components:
   - *Deflecting lever*: Based on the direction of deflection of the tip of ureteroscope with respect to the direction of movement of deflecting lever, the deflection mechanism has been classified into two types.

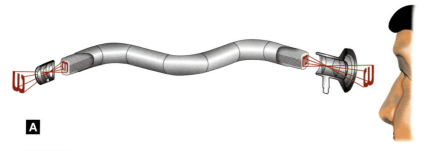

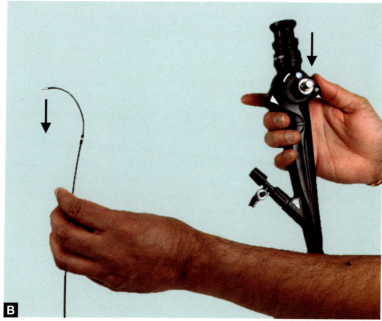

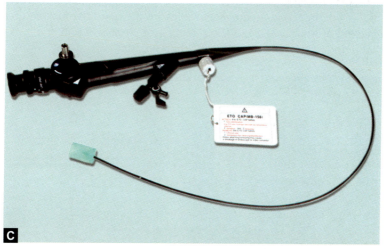

Figures 1A to C: (A) Schematic representation of flexible ureteroscopes; (B) Logic type flexible ureteroscope; (C) Flexible ureteroscope

In logic (intuitive, positive or American) type, direction of deflection of tip corresponds to that of the lever, i.e. down is down and up is up. In anti-logic (counter-intuitive, contrapositive or European) type, direction of deflection of tip is opposite to that of the lever.

- *Working channel*: Working channel is used to insert graspers, baskets, wires and laser fibers. The inner diameter of working channel is 3.6 Fr. This allows the use of instruments of size up to 3 Fr with concurrent irrigation. Irrigation port is connected to the working channel port at a right angle.
- *Seal*: The seal is fitted on the inlet channel. The device consists of a O-ring that fits the size of the instruments inserted into the working channel. It prevents loss of irrigation fluid around the instrument and can be used to fix the laser fiber at a particular distance from the tip of the instrument.
- *Light post*: The fiberoptic light cable is attached to the light post.

3. *Shaft*: The shaft encases fiberoptic bundles for image and light transmission, working channel and wires for deflection mechanism. The size of flexible ureteroscope is quoted by its tip diameter, which is 7.5 Fr in the case of Storz flex X2. The working length of the instrument is 67 cm and working channel is 3.6 Fr. The shock absorbing system is a form of secondary deflection, which is present in modern flexible ureteroscopes. It is located proximal to the active deflecting system and allows for gentle rolling of the distal end for approximately ten centimeters enabling access more deeply into the calyces (Figure 2).

4. *Tip*: The objective lens is made of 2–9 lenses as well as a prism if different viewing directions are required. No prism is required if the viewing angle is 0°. It changes the incident light into an image, projecting it onto the image guide.

The tip has the distal ends of fiberoptic bundles carrying image to camera and light from the light source. The distal end of working channel opens below the fiberoptic bundles. The 1.5 cm laserite™ ceramic-coated tip at the distal end of the working channel prevents thermal damage to the flexible ureterorenoscope during laser usage.[1] The direction of view is 0° and angle of view is 88°. The tip can be deflected 270° in either direction.

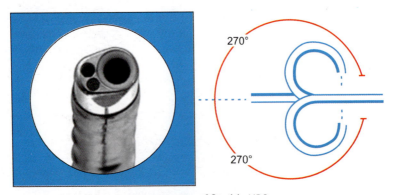

Figure 2: Tip of flexible URS

Why Dual Deflection has Disappeared?

The primary purpose of dual deflection was to improve access to lower pole calyces. The older flexible ureteroscopes had a primary deflection angle less than 200°. Dual deflection mechanism achieves a deflection angle around 300° by deflecting the scope at two places. Newer ureteroscopes have a larger deflection angle with a single deflection mechanism, which allows easy entry into lower calyces. Moreover, dual deflection levers are more cumbersome to use.

What do you mean by Active and Passive Deflection?

When the tip of the flexible ureteroscope is deflected using the deflecting lever, which controls the tip through wires, it is called active deflection. When the tip of the flexible ureteroscope bends against the wall of the pelvis to enter the calyx, especially the lower calyx, it is called passive deflection.

	Tip diameter (Fr)	Shaft diameter (Fr)	Working length (cm)	Working channel (Fr)	Active deflection up (degree)	Active deflection down (degree)	Angle of view (degree)	Field of view (degree)
Fiberoptic								
Flex X2	7.5	8.4	67.5	3.6	270	270	0	88
URF P6	4.9	7.95	67	3.6	275	275	0	90
Wolf Viper	6	8.8	68	3.6	270	270	0	86
Wolf Cobra	6	9.9	68	3.3 x 2	270	270	0	86
ACMI DUR 8E	6.75	8.6	64	3.6	170	180 (130 secondary active deflection)	9	80
Digital								
Flex Xc	8.5	8.4	70	3.6	270	270	0	90
Olympus	8.5	9.9	67	3.6	180	275	0	90
Invisio D-URD	8.7	9.3	65	3.6	250	250	0	80

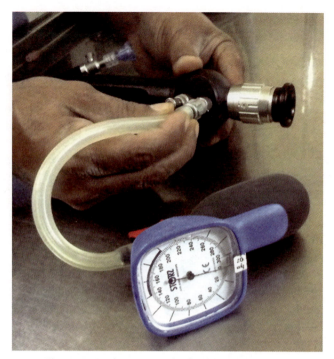

Figure 3: Leakage tester for flexible ureteroscopy

What is Leakage Tester?

Leakage tester is used to verify the integrity of the flexible ureteroscope's working channel. The leakage tester is connected to the special port located at the body of the ureteroscope and scope is pressurized about 140–200 mm Hg by pumping the bulb. Monitor the indicator to detect any fall in pressure, which indicates a leak (Figure 3).

Comparison of the Currently Available Flexible Ureteroscopes

Evolution of Flexible Ureteroscopes

The use of a flexible ureteroscope (9 Fr) was first reported by Marshall in 1964.[2] In 1970s a cystoscopically placed guide tube into the ureter (access sheath) was developed to allow flow of irrigation fluid around the instrument to improve visibility. In the 1980s, irrigation channel and a working channel were combined and incorporated into the next generation of ureteroscopes along with an active deflection mechanism. ACMI DUR8 ureteroscope had an upward deflection angle of 175° and downward deflection angle of 185°. With this angle of deflection, it was difficult to enter lower pole calyces that were highly angulated. Then, ACMI DUR8 Elite was introduced with a secondary active deflection of 130° controlled by a second lever. Then, newer ureteroscopes with better primary angle of defection (e.g. Flex X2) were developed. The most recent development is the availability of digital ureteroscopes with clear, magnified image and better depth perception (e.g. Flex Xc).

Parts of Digital Flexible Ureteroscopes

1. *Body*: The body is attached to an integrated cable containing wires to carry electronic signals of image and fiberoptic bundles to carry light. It has a working channel port and deflection lever. In contrast to fiberoptic scopes, there is no focusing component.
2. *Shaft*: The shaft has a slightly larger diameter than those of fiberoptic ureteroscopes.
3. *Tip*: The tip design of Flex- Xc has a working channel below the objective lens in the middle. The light bundles are divided into two and end on either side of the objective lens. This provides more uniform lighting in the operative field.

How does a Digital Flexible Ureteroscope Differ from a Fiberoptic Ureteroscope?

In a digital flexible ureteroscope, the image is captured by the camera sensor at the tip of the ureteroscope just behind the objective lens. This image is carried as electronic signals through wires. In a fiberoptic system, the image from objective lens is carried by fiberoptic bundles to the eyepiece.

What is 'Chip on the Tip' Principle?

In chip on tip, the ureteroscope tip itself contains a camera sensor. The image generated in the objective lens is projected onto to the video chip, which converts the optical signals into electrical signals and transmits them to the camera controller. With the chip on tip there is superior appreciation of depth of field and no need for focusing.

The two different technologies used for capturing images digitally are: CCD (charge coupled device) and CMOS (complementary metal oxide semiconductor) image sensors. In a CCD sensor, every pixel's charge is transferred through an output nodes to be converted to voltage, buffered, and sent off-chip as an analog signal. All of the pixel can be devoted to light capture, and the output's uniformity is high. In a CMOS sensor, each pixel has its own charge-to-voltage conversion, and the sensor often includes amplifiers, noise-correction, and digitization circuits, so that the chip outputs digital bits. These other functions increase the design complexity and reduce the area available for light capture. With each pixel doing its own conversion, uniformity is lower.

Advantages of Digital Flexible Ureteroscope

The image transfer is better since the chip at the tip directly receives it. Image quality is equivalent to ten times the pixel resolution of standard fiberoptic endoscopes. Since there is no need for attaching a camera, the instrument becomes light and easy to manipulate. The wear and tear is lower as there is no fiberoptic bundle in this ureteroscope.

Disadvantages of Digital Flexible Ureteroscope

Since tip size increases because of chip at the tip, patients require more ureteric dilatation with larger access sheaths and there is an increased chance of staging the procedure if ureter could not be adequately dilated. Even the smallest digital flexible ureteroscope is 8.5 Fr in size. Further, these ureteroscopes are more expensive.

Accessories (See Chapter on Accessories)

Various accessories required are:
1. Access sheath.
2. Wires-Bi wire, glide wires.
3. Baskets-engage, entrap, etc.
4. Laser fiber.

REFERENCES

1. Online catalog of Karl Storz. Uretero-renoscopes Flex-X2 and Flex-X, 9th edition, 2012, pp. 202-4. Website. http://epc.karlstorz.com/epc/Starter.jsp?locale=EN&practiceArea=URO&product=&sid=SID-E02F3390-37621460. Accessed on 20th July 2013.
2. Marshall VF. Fiber optics in urology. J Urol. 1964;91:110-4.

Laparoscopy and Robotics: Instruments

LAPAROSCOPIC INSTRUMENTS

Introduction and Brief History

The first laparoscopic nephrectomy was performed by Clayman in 1991.[1] The first laparoscopic donor nephrectomy was performed by Ratner[2] Rane and colleagues are credited with the first urologic laparoendoscopic single-site (LESS) surgery.[3]

In this chapter, we describe the various instruments required for laparoscopic and robotic surgery. The instruments are described with emphasis on their specifications and uses.

The laparoscopic instruments will be described as follows:
1. Armamentarium required for urologic laparoscopy.
2. Access related instruments. (Veress needle)
3. Trocars.
4. Laparoscopic dissecting and retracting instruments.
5. Laparoscopic telescopes.
6. Clips applicator and staplers.

The Armamentarium

Proper instruments are the 'key' to successful completion of the procedure. Prior to initiating the procedure the surgeon should prepare a checklist as well as make sure that all the required instruments are arranged in a systematic manner on the operating room trolley. The instruments will vary as per the case, however, the general outline of armamentarium required for laparoscopy includes the following:
1. Camera unit (Sterilizable head and cable, video control unit).
2. Connector cables from camera to monitor.
3. Video monitor.
4. Light source.
5. Light transmission fiberoptic cable.
6. Insufflators.
7. Carbon dioxide cylinder.
8. Carbon dioxide pressure regulator valve.

9. Tubing and Luer-lock adapter for carbon dioxide to patient.
10. Suction irrigation apparatus.
11. Cautery machine with cables and foot control.
12. Extension cord.
13. Telescope.
14. Trocars and cannulas.
15. Veress needle.
16. Atraumatic graspers.
17. Toothed grasper.
18. Curved dissector.
19. Clip applicator with suitable clips.
20. Dissection hook.
21. Laparoscopic scissors.
22. Suction irrigation cannula.
23. Laparoscopic needle holder.

The trolley is arranged in systematic fashion, and the telescope white balanced. Preferably the assistant should be trained in this aspect. The surgical principles remain the same in arranging the trolley as in open surgery. Sharp instruments should be kept away from the field, telescopes and cameras are placed in the center of the trolley and properly secured. A rescue tray at all times should be kept ready on the table. The rescue tray includes:

1. Needle which is prepared with a hem-o-lok™ clip attached to the tail of the needle (Rescue stitch). Typically a rescue stitch is a stitch on a CT1 needle with a hem-o-lok™ clip attached to the tail end of the suture. A knot is thrown over the hem-o-lok clip to prevent its slippage.
2. A hemostatic agent such as surgicel™.
3. A cartridge of vascular clip such as hem-o-lok™ clip.
4. A gauze which can be easily inserted through the port and has a radiopaque marker.
5. Two needle holders.
6. Satinsky clamp.

The rescue stitch should be placed in a readily visible part of the operating room (OR) and used in the event of life-threatening bleeding.

Access Devices

The access devices will vary with the approach (Trans or retro). Proper peritoneal access is crucial for successful completion of surgery. Pneumoperitoneum can be achieved either with closed or open technique. The open technique is known as 'Hassans technique'. The advantages of the open technique include, theoretical less chance of bowel injury, however if the fascial incision exceeds the diameter of the port it may cause gas leak.

Insufflation Devices

- *Veress needle (Figure 1)*: The veress needle is available either as a disposable or reusable needle. These are manufactured by Storz, Wolf as well as a few

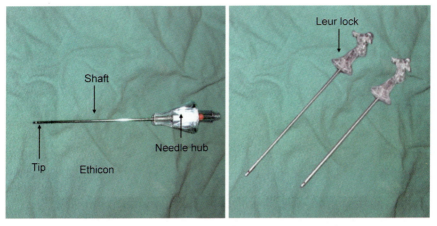

Figure 1: The Autosuture and Ethicon veress needles

Indian manufacturers. Disposable veress needles are manufactured by Autosuture, and Ethicon.

Veress needle is available in three lengths 80 mm, 100 mm, 120 mm. The length is measured from the tip to the hub. The longer one is useful in obese patients (150 mm). It is 14 gauge in diameter. The reusable needle is larger in diameter (3 mm).

The veress needle has three parts (Figure 2)

1. *The hub*: The hub of the veress needle has an indicator which suggests the position of the needle (preperitoneal or peritoneal), a green indicator indicates the tip of the needle is in a negative milieu (peritoneum), a red indicator indicates the tip is in a preperitoneal space or is in the mesenteric fat or the needle is blocked (This feature is seen in Ethicon needle, not seen in autosuture). This is safety mechanism, once the inner component completely protrudes beyond the stylet, the green indicator will show up, indicating it is in a hollow cavity, even with a minimal resistance (partially in), it will show up as a red indicator. The floating ball (red or green) at the center of the hub, will float when the tip of the needle is in the peritoneum. The hub has a leur lock arrangement, which helps to attach syringe, thereby confirming the presence of needle in peritoneal cavity, on aspiration of air it confirms presence of needle in the desired cavity. The floating ball remains suspended in the cylindrical portion of the hub, as the needle enters the peritoneal space, the ball falls to the base of the cylindrical space of the hub.
2. *The shaft*: It is metallic and is radiopaque. The shaft provides a conduit for passage of gas for insufflations.
3. *The tip*: The tip has two components. The inner component is blunt and projects just beyond the tip of the sharp needle (for 3 mm). The sharp needle (outer beveled sheath) helps in penetration of the needle across the fascia into the peritoneal cavity, once the needle enters the negative milieu of the peritoneum, the sharp tip retracts, this helps in preventing injury to

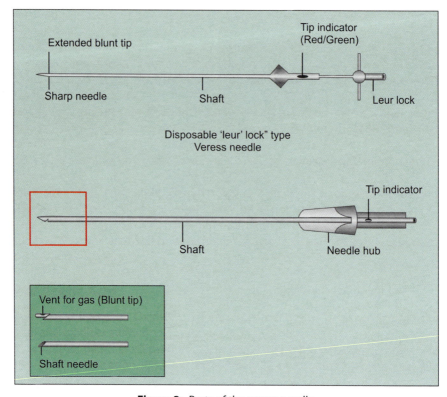

Figure 2: Parts of the veress needle

the intraperitoneal organs. The lateral hole (opposite to the bevel) on the needle enables CO_2 to be delivered intra-abdominally. When the hole is inside the outer sheath insufflations does not occur, hence theoretically preventing subcutaneous emphysema.

While inserting it should be held like a dart. It is important to check the patency and the spring action of the Veress needle.

Types of Trocars (Figure 3)

The trocars offer a conduit for entry and exit of instruments during the surgery. The trocars are available in various sizes ranging from 2 mm to 15 mm. The operating surgeon needs to understand the instruments which need to be passed through a suitably sized port.

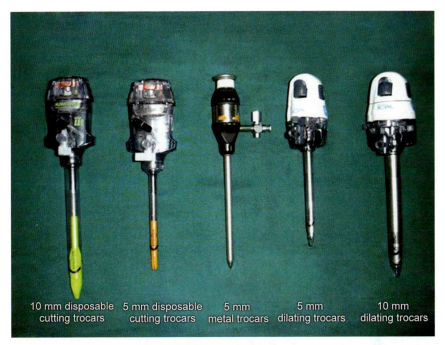

10 mm disposable cutting trocars | 5 mm disposable cutting trocars | 5 mm metal trocars | 5 mm dilating trocars | 10 mm dilating trocars

Figure 3: The trocars classification

The trocars can be classified in the following ways:
- Disposable (plastic)
- Nondisposable (metal) (Figure 6).

They can also be classified as:
- Bladed trocars
- Nonbladed trocars.

They can also be classified depending on size—commonly used are 5 mm, 11 mm and 12 mm.

Special types of trocar:
- *Miniport (Ethicon) (Figure 4B)*: The port has two parts, an outer hollow sheath which acts a port, the Veress needle can be inserted through the outer sheath.
- Hybrid trocars (Autosuture) (both 5 mm and 11 mm channel) (Figure 4A). It has two channels one for 10 mm and second for 5 mm.
- *Newer smudge port (Ethicon)*: The specially designed valve prevents smudge and fogging of the telescope.

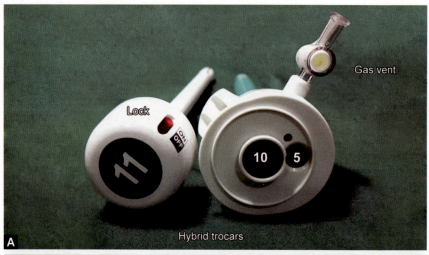

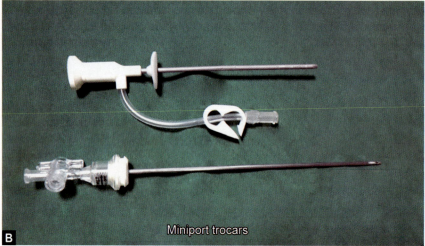

Figures 4A and B: The port has two parts, a outer hollow sheath which acts a port, the Veress needle can be inserted through the outer sheath

The trocar assembly (disposable) consists of (Figure 5):
The parts are: Cannula, obturator (trocar) and reducer.
Cannula: Cannula is made from plastic or metal. It has a shaft and housing. The shaft length is measured from the beveled length to housing. The shaft length and size is available as 75 mm (short) (only in 5 mm), 100 mm (standard) (12 mm, 5 mm) and 150 mm (extra long) (12, 5 mm). The cannula tip can be either straight or oblique. The parts of housing include valve and a gas vent with stop cock. The gas vent is distal to the valve. The valves in disposable trocars are nonflap, while in reusable trocars they are of a trumpet (flap) configuration. The housing also features a knob for attaching the reducer. The valves of cannula provide internal air seals, which allow instruments to move

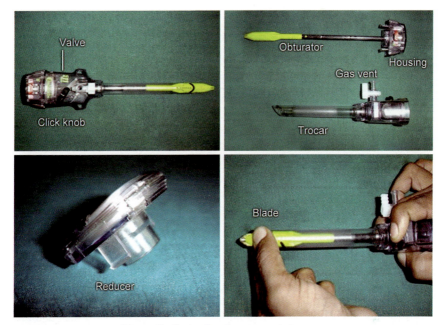

Figure 5: Parts of an laparoscopic trocars

in and out within the cannula without the loss of pneumoperitoneum. These valves can be oblique, transverse, or in piston configuration. The valves can be manually or automatically retractable during instrument passage after removing the reducer.

Reducers (Figure 5): It is used to reduce the size of the port from 11, 12, 10 mm to 5 mm, so that pneumoperitoneum is maintained, whenever surgeon changes the instrument from larger diameter to smaller diameter. The reducer sheaths are available either as (hollow rods) or can be used as attachments which can be fixed on the housing of the trocars.

Universal Reducer

Port size specific reducer (10, 11, 15, 5), No reducer for 5 mm.

Obturator: The obturator can be bladed or nonbladed. The obturator can be optiview (transparent at tip of trocar) or nonoptiview. The obturator has a knob/lock for attachment to the cannula while it has lateral knob for fixation of the telescope. All cannulas have a end hole through which a appropriate size telescope can be passed. The obturator of disposable trocars has a sharp blade which retracts as soon as the trocar passes through the abdominal wall. The blade protrudes on resistance to tough tissue and retracts (unlocked) in negative milieu. The bladed trocars can be used as nonbladed provided you do not load the blade. The bladed disposable trocars are not freely available.

Reusable Trocars

Hassan trocar: The Hassan's cannula offers the advantage of reduced risk of injury to the bowels. It is especially useful in a patient who has previously undergone intra-abdominal procedures.

Parts of the cannula:
This cannula consists of three pieces:
1. A cone-shaped sleeve.
2. A metal or plastic sheath with a trumpet or flap valve (Figure 6). The sheath has two struts for affixing fascial sutures. These sutures are then wrapped tightly around the struts. Thereby firmly seating the cone-shaped sleeve into the laparoscopic port. This creates an effective seal to maintain pneumoperitoneum.
3. Blunt tipped obturator.

Instruments Used for the Retroperitoneal Approach

Dr Gaur is credited with the description of new device/technique for retroperitoneal surgery.[4] The retroperitoneal space is developed initially with the finger till the thoracolumbar fascia, once this is pierced either with a finger or a instrument the space is created with a custom-made dissector or a glove and inflated with a rubber catheter. Alternatively a balloon is available which helps in creation of the retroperitoneal space.

Retracting and Dissecting Instruments

The retractors are either disposable or nondisposable. The nondisposable instruments can be dismantled, so that they can be cleaned and reused.
The parts of the instruments are (Figure 7):
1. Handle.
2. Insulated outer tube.
3. Inner tube which is part of the tip of the instrument.

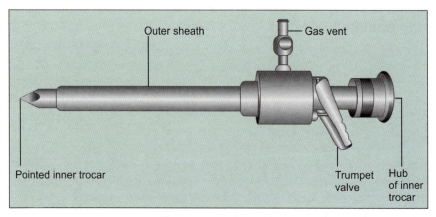

Figure 6: Metal cannula

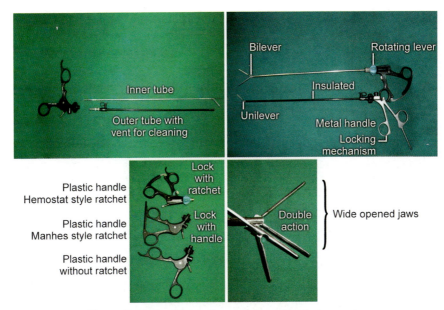

Figure 7: Parts of retracting and dissecting instruments

The design and mechanism of action for the handle, outer sheath and inner sheath differs with manufacturers.

1. *Insulated outer tube*: The outer tube may be insulated or noninsulated. Insulation covering may be of silicon or plastic. The insulation coat is likely to be breached during cleaning and may be dangerous as this may lead to inadvertent injury during the course of surgery. The surgeon should make sure that the insulation cover is not breached prior to commencing the surgery. The outer tube also has a vent for cleaning and sterilizing. This helps to clean the instrument without dismantling the instrument. This feature is not seen in wolf outer sheath. Extra long outer sheath is 42 cm in length.

2. *Insert of the instrument (Figure 8)*: The insert of the instrument can be a scissor, grasper or forceps, Maryland, Allis, etc. As shown in the figure, the forceps or the grasper will be a single action mechanism or a double action mechanism. The jaws of the single action grasper open less than double action grasper. The single action graspers exert more force between the jaws than the double action. The double action is used for retraction while single action is for grasping. The insert is locked by rotating the distal end and clicking on the lock.

Storz instrument handle: This can be plastic or metal.

The parts of the handle are:

1. Finger grip.
2. Rotating knob.
3. Release button to release the inner and outer sheath.
4. Cautery attachment.

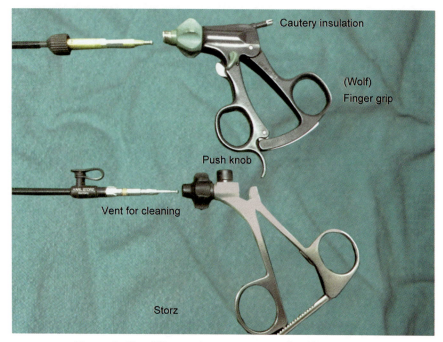

Figure 8: The difference between storz and wolf instrument

Handle: The handle of the 'hand held' laparoscopic instruments have either a locking or nonlocking mechanism. The handle also has a pillar for attaching the cautery cable. The locking mechanism includes a 'ratchet' mechanism for locking (Storz) or a button mechanism (Wolf) (Figure 8). The locking mechanism helps the surgeon to maintain the instrument in a fixed position and hence avoids fatigue in prolonged surgeries. Most of the laparoscopic instruments handle have attachments for unipolar electrosurgical lead and many have rotator mechanism to rotate the tip of the instrument. The cautery attachment is oblique to the shaft. The latter arrangement may cause clashing which is avoided in a cautery pillar placed in a coaxial manner. The finger grip has special grooves for adjusting fingers.

The Press knob on the handle is a feature of storz instrument. The wolf instruments does not have press knob.

Types of Ratchet for Retracting Instruments

1. Manhes style ratchet (Storz catalogue 33122).
2. Hemostat style ratchet (Storz catalogue 33123).
3. Disengageable ratchet (Storz catalogue 33126).

Fan Retractor

The parts of a fan retractor are:
1. Outer tube -5 Fr and 10 Fr.
2. The inner tube has a grip and fans which get retracted inside the outer tube in resting position. It has 9 fan blades.

Needle Holders (Figure 9)

The needle holder has either a pistol grip or straight grip. The grip is always single action as it offers a firm grip of the needle. The tip of the needle holder may be curved (right curve or left curve) or straight. The needle holders varies in length (33 cm). The pediatric needle holder is shorter in length (23 cm). In-line grip needle holders are ergonomically better than pistol grip needle holder.

Parts of the Needle Driver

Generally they cannot be dismantled, laparoscopic needle holders are always locking. The lock can be thumb lock or finger lock. The needle driver can be single toothed.

The parts are as follows:
- *Tip*: Curved (right or left), straight.
- *Shaft*: It has a cleaning vent.
- *Handle*: The handle can be pistol grip or a inline grip.

KOH Macro needle holders. This is manufactured by Storz GmBH. It can be disassembled into the following parts namely.
1. The handle.
2. Working insert.
3. Outer tube. The inserts are made of tungsten carbide.

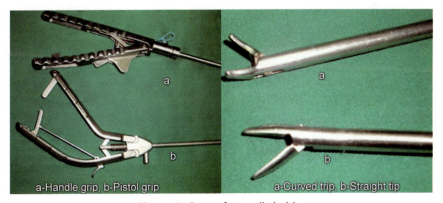

a-Handle grip, b-Pistol grip   a-Curved trip, b-Straight tip

Figure 9: Parts of a needle holder

Laparoscopic Scissors (Figures 10A and B)

The type of scissors used varies according to the purpose of use and the surgeon comfort. The laparoscopic scissors can be used as a cold shears or hot shears.

Parts of the Scissors

In reusable scissors, the parts mimic those of retracting instruments, in the sense it can be dismantled into insert, outer tube and handle. The disposable scissors is integrated. These instruments are 30 cm in length.
They can be classified as:
1. Disposable.
2. Nondisposable.

Laparoscopic scissors can also be classified as:
1. *Straight scissors*: They are available either as short jaws or long jaw scissors. The longer straight variety is useful when performing donor nephrectomy to achieve optimal length of the vessels. The short straight scissors can be used as an aid during suturing.
2. *Curved shears*: They can be used as dissectors. These are useful in spatulation of the ureter, during ureteric reimplantation, or pyeloplasty. During spatulation of a pyeloplasty, the ureter can be rotated inline with the instrument, the left hand is used for spatulation of the left ureter and scissors in the right hand for spatulation of the right sided ureter. Long straight scissors can be used during partial nephrectomy as it delivers long cuts hence restricting warm ischemia time.
3. *Roticulator scissors*: The tip of the scissors rotates on its axis, this helps in spatulation during pyeloplasty and ureteric reimplantation.

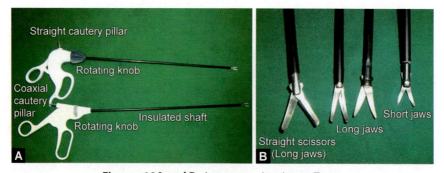

Figures 10A and B: Laparoscopic scissors: Types

Clip Applicators and Staplers

The clip applicators can be classified as:
1. Preloaded (example—Ligamax™, Allport™)
2. Nonpreloaded with additional cartridge (example—Hem-o-lok™).

They can be also classified as:
1. Multiload (example—Allport™ Ligamax™)
2. Single load (example—Titanium clips)

They also can be classified as:
1. Disposable
2. Multiple use.

The clips that were initially used were multiple use and single load, the disadvantages were additional time required for every load, clips used to accidentally fall off while passing through the trocars and they lacked a rotating handle. All these shortcomings are overcome with multiload clips.

The advantages of multiload clips are:
1. 360° rotating shafts.
2. Clips do not fall off while passing through the trocars.
3. Saves time while loading.

They can also be classified as:
1. Noninterlocking titanium clips 200 (white), 300 (green) and 400 (yellow)
2. Polymer clips (Hem-o-lok clips) green (medium), (violet) large medium and (gold) extra large.

The color code is for the clip applicator and color code knob is located on the clip applicator. The clip applicator assembly includes the applicator and the clips. The varieties of clips available commonly used are Hem-o-lok™ and Ligaclip™. The other clips available are Ligaclip™, Ligamax™.

Hem-o-lok Clip Applicators (Teleflex Medical Inc)

This is a nonabsorbable polymer clip. There were concerns with the application of the Hem-o-lok clips in donor nephrectomy. A FDA warning (www.fda.gov/ Medwatch/report.htm) has contraindicated the use of hem-o-lok clips in laparoscopic donor nephrectomy. The hem-o-lok clips are made of polymer and are radiolucent. They are available as a cartridge of 6 clips. They are interlocking clips and are held securely with the help of a knob and lock mechanism. The hem-o-lok clips are available in three sizes namely XL-gold, L-purple and S-white (Figure 11). A multi institutional working group compiled a retrospective review of laparoscopic procedures in 9 institutions. The procedures reviewed included 899 radical nephrectomies, 112 simple nephrectomies, 198 nephroureterectomies and 486 donor nephrectomies. No clips failed in this series.[5]

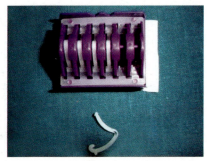

Figure 11: L-sizeclip color code is purple

Hem-o-lok Clip Applicator (Figure 12)

This device is autoclavable, reusable. It cannot be dismantled.
The parts of hem-o-lok clip applicators are:
- *Handle:* The handle has a palm grip and a thumb grip. The finger grip moves while the palm is fixed and provides support.
- *Rotator:* This features the color code of the clips to be applied. It helps in rotating the jaws. The shaft connects the handle to the tip and the jaws. The shaft has a vent for cleaning and sterilization.
- *Tip/Jaw:* The jaw features a knob which corresponds to the knob on the clip. The jaws make a angle of approximately 5–10 degree to the shaft. This helps in application of the clips to the lumbar, gonadal and adrenal vein.

How to Load the Clips?

Rules
- The clip applicator should be held at 90° to the handle of the clip.
- This should ensure that the knob fits into the corresponding notch on the tip of the jaw and the handle of the clip fits into the groove.

Hem-o-lok™ Clip: Rules for Application (Figure 13)

1. Always circumferentially dissect the vessel in concern prior to application.
2. Hear the click of the knob after application of the clip.
3. Always see the knob of the clip prior to application.

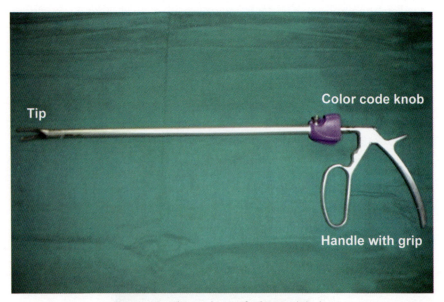

Figure 12: Clip applicator for hem-o-lok clip

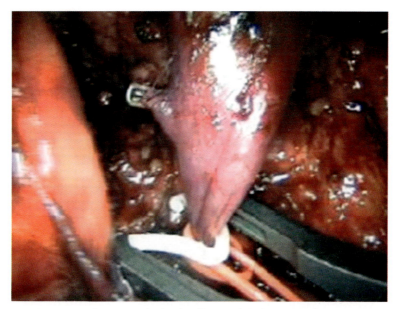

Figure 13: Always see the knob of hem-o-lok clip prior to application

4. Always apply two clips on the patient side.
5. At least leave 2 mm cuff beyond the cut end of the clip.[5]

Hem-o-lok clips can be removed as follows:
- Hem-o-lok™ clip remover.
- The clip can be cut open with harmonic scalpel.

Interlocking metal clips (also called as biting clips) (Allport™ Ethicon Endosurgery Inc Cincinnati OH, Ligamax™, Ligaclip) (Ethicon Endosurgery Inc OH), Endoclip (Autosuture, US surgical, Norwalk, CT). These clips are radiopaque and are interlocking, they are useful in securing smaller vessels such as the adrenal vein and the lumbar veins. They can be removed on the backbench and hence are useful in donor nephrectomy. These clips come preloaded and have clips in the set of 12–20. Ligamax™ (15 clips multiload). All these have a one time use/one patient use feature.

The typical preloaded clip applicator has the following components:
- *Handle*: The handle features an indicator which indicates the amount of clips consumed (The indicator color changes from white to orange as the clips get consumed). The finger grip gets locked once all the clips in the preloaded cartridge are consumed.
- *Shaft*: The length of the shaft is 32 cm (Ligamax™)
- *Tip*: The tip of a preloaded clip applicator has two metal jaws. Both the jaws move. Once the clip is deployed through the shaft the clip is simultaneously further deployed in between the jaws. The jaws are capable of movement on a 360° axis.

Types of Interlocking Clips (Figure 14)

- *Ligaclip™ allport*: This is manufactured by ethicon endosurgery, it is compatible with port size of 5 mm. It is available in a cartridge of 20–30 clips. It is available as medium, medium large or large sizes. The clip loading is automatic.
- *Ligaclip™ right angle*: It is manufactured by Ethicon Endosurgery, it is compatible with port size of 10 mm. It is available in a cartridge of 20 clips. It is available as medium-large sizes. The clip loading is automatic.
- *Ligaclip™ MCA*: It is manufactured by Ethicon Endosurgery, it is compatible with port size of 12 mm. It is available in a cartridge of 20 clips. It is available as large size. The clip loading is automatic.
- *Endoclip™*: Manufactured by Autosuture. It is compatible with port size of 5 mm It is available in a cartridge of 20 clips. It is available as medium-large size. The clip loading is with separate lever.
- *Endoclip™ II*: Manufactured by Autosuture. It is compatible with port size of 10 mm. It is available in a cartridge of 20 clips. It is available as medium-large and large size. The clip loading is automatic.
- *Endoclip™ multapplier*: Manufactured by Autosuture. It is compatible with port size of 10 mm. It is available in a cartridge of 8 clips. It is available as medium-large and large size. The clip loading is automatic.

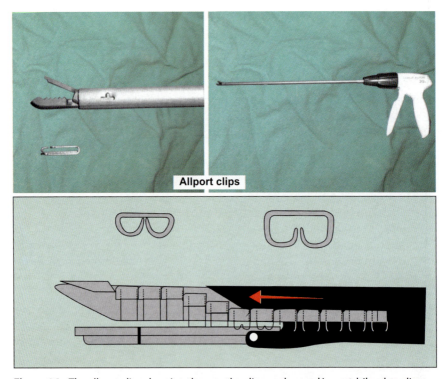

Allport clips

Figure 14: The allport clips showing the way the clips are housed in a multiload applicator

Laparoscopic Staplers[6]

Broadly the staplers can be classified as:
1. Circular.
2. Linear.
3. Linear cutting.
4. Ligating.

The linear staplers can be further classified as:
1. *Cutting*: Six parallel rows of staples are fired. Once this is fired a knife follows which leaves three staplers on either side. Always the staple line extends beyond the cut edge to avoid leaving any nonsecured edge. The knife cannot be redeployed without reloading the stapler.
2. *Noncutting staplers*: These staplers simply fire four rows of staples and are helpful in right sided donor nephrectomies for gaining extra length of the vein and repairing bladder injuries.

The staplers can also be classified by length of staple line

30/35, 45 and 60 mm. Further they can be classified depending on weather the firing end is articulating or otherwise. All the staplers have a rotating shaft. A stapling device has the following main components (Figure 15).

1. *Cartridge*: They are further classified depending on length of the cartridge (30, 45 and 60 mm.

    Cartridges are color coded. White cartridge is for vascular stapling and blue is for other tissues. White is meant for compression of tissues to less than 1 mm whereas blue is meant for tissue compression to less than 1.5 mm.
2. *Shaft*: Shaft can be straight or articulating.
3. *Handle*: It has two or three parts and has an additional button which during use will first put suturing staples and later between the staple lines it will put incision and cut.

    Recently power staplers are available which are automated and use the battery energy for above actions.

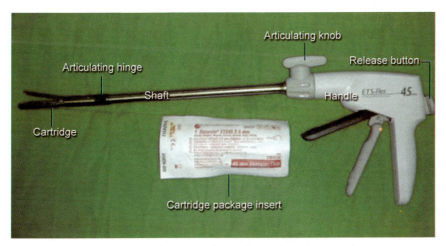

Figure 15: Parts of a stapler

Miscellaneous Instruments

1. *Sottelotome*: It is an instrument with working length of 42 cm with 5 mm diameter. It has spatulated end which is curved and measures 6 cm in length. It has rounded nontraumatic tip. It is useful for delivering stone during laparoscopic pyelolithotomy, nephrolithotomy as well as during hilar dissection, single port transvesical prostatectomy.
2. *Laparoscopic satinsky forceps*: It is 10 mm in diameter and has 40 cm length. Jaw length is 7 cm. It also has cleaning port for instrument cleaning. It is available as single action or double action, i.e. either only one or both the jaws are mobile.
3. *Probe plus II (Ethicon Endosurgery, OH)*: This instrument is used for laparoscopic stone surgery. The components of this instrument include:
   – *Handle*: The handle has a two button one for suction and one for irrigation. It also has a corresponding tubing for suction and irrigation ports. The handle also has a monopolar cautery attachment. The hub of the handle has a red button for detaching the shaft/probe. The probe rotates on its own axis.

   The probe has a outer covering and inner insert. The outer covering features a knob for rotating the probe and a cannula which helps in performing suction and irrigation at the distal end.

   The inner insert is available in two types:
   i. *Needle tip*: Used for incising the pelvis and the ureter
   ii. *Spatula tip*: Used for dislodging the calculus. The insert can be retracted in and out and helps in precise control.
4. Bull dog clip applier:

   The parts of the instrument are:
   • *Handle*: It has a finger grip and a thumb grip. In addition, it also has a knob (lock) for applying and releasing the bull dog clamp.
   • The shaft is self-rotating and has a cleaning vent. The tip of the applier has a knob which gets fixed with the socket of the bull dog clamp.
   • *Laparoscopic telescopes*: The telescopes can be classified depending on angle of view, size (5 mm, 10 mm), rigid or flexitip, and length of telescope (long and short) and coaxial and noncoaxial.

Angle of View (Figure 16)

Three varieties of telescopes are available. They include zero degree, thirty degree and Forty five degree.

1. *Zero degree lens*: It is a straight lens and typically used in operations on the pelvis. These operations include those on the prostate, bladder and the lower ureter. The color code of these lens is green. The method of sterilization is autoclavable. Light transmission is through fiberoptic cables. Image transmission is through rod lens (H_2). They are available as 10 mm and 5 mm. Although longer telescopes are available the usual length is 33 cm (working length) (total 39 cm: eyepeice to tip).

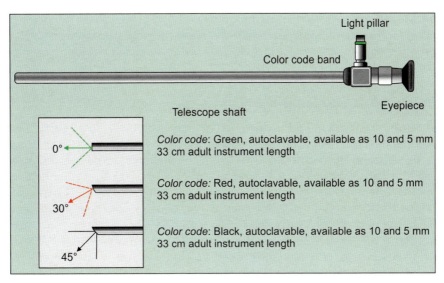

Figure 16: Laparoscopes: Angle of view

2. *Thirty degree lens*: This lens which has a color code red is used, the length is 33 cm. They are sterilized with an autoclave. The lens is typically used in surgeries on the kidney as the lens helps in visualizing the posterior aspect of renal hilum.
3. *Forty five degree lens*: The use of these telescopes is not common color code is black, 33 cm in length.

Special Laparoscopes

1. *Coaxial cable laparoscopes*: The Olympus endoeye™ has a coaxial light cable. It is particularly useful in single site surgery as the light pillar of the routinely used camera produces a 'nutcracker' effect because of clashing of instruments. The coaxial light cable helps in preventing clashing. A few variations in this laparoscope are available which include laparoscopes with an extender and a flexible tip laparoscope, both these variations are helpful in preventing crowding and clashing of instruments.
2. *Endocameleon*: This telescope has a feature of having a interchangeable angle of view (0–120). The angle of view can be decided according to the procedure to be done and surgeon preference.
3. *3D laparoscopes*: These laparoscopes give a 3D vision. The surgical field has to be viewed with 3D glasses.
4. *Needloscopes*: Can be introduced through a miniport or a Veress needle.

ROBOTICS SURGERY IN UROLOGY

The use of robotic assisted laparoscopic surgery has increased exponentially over the past few decades across various surgical disciplines. Initially targeted for cardiac applications, the use in urology is what proved to be the tipping point for its current popularity. There are many theoretical advantages of the robotic surgical system which include 3D, HD vision improved dexterity, tremor filtration.

Equipments and Supplies

The basic requirement for the operating room is, it should be large enough to accommodate all the components of the robot. The various items which need to be procured beyond those available in the operating room are; reusable robotic accessories such as sterile drapes, scopes (0° and 30°), light guide cables, specific 8 mm robotic instrument compatible trocars. The hospital needs to decide the inventory prior to commencement of cases. The other equipment which are needed are a suction/irrigator, scope warmer, a surgeon chair with a optimal height so that the surgeon can see comfortably in the console, video equipment for recording. To say it in short, robotics is 'labor intensive'. A dedicated team is essential. A constantly changing team might hamper the program from an efficacy and result standpoint.

The components of the robot include a patient cart, a vision cart and the console. The surgeon sits on the console and controls the masters. The currently available robot is known as the *Da Vinci Si*, The previous two generations were *Da Vinci* and *Da Vinci S*.

The patient cart has the following components:

The central pillar and the patient safety manipulator (PSM). The arms work on the principle of remote center technology wherein the arms move around a fixed point in space and provide the expected dexterity and precision.

Robotic Instrumentation (Figure 17)

- *Robotic trocars*: These are reusable and are available with reducers. The shaft of the trocars has a black band which is known as the 'remote center'. After insertion of the port the band should lie on the inner surface of the perito- neum. This band acts as a remote point in space around which the robotic arms move. The robotic ports can be sterilized with autoclave or plasma sterilization. The robotic trocars are available as 8 mm and 5 mm trocars.
- *Robotic drapes*: These are one time use drapes which have adapter to be installed on the robotic arms.
- *Robotic working instruments*: They are robotic shears, robotic needle holder, robotic Maryland (bipolar forceps), robotic scissors, robotic hook, all these instruments have a limited use depending on whether they are training instruments, or pediatric use instruments.

The parts of typical robotic instrument are as follows. The only contraindication for its use are its use on cartilage, bone and hard objects.

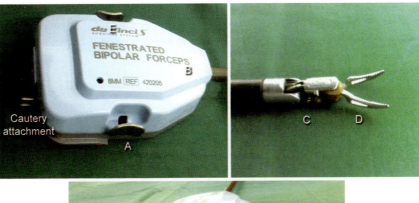

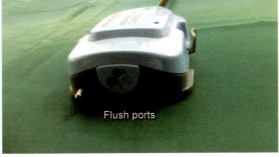

Figure 17: The release lever (A), the instrument shaft (B), the wrist (C), tip or end effector (D) instrument housing (E)

These instruments are called as endowrist instrument™. The five main components:

- The release lever (A)
- The instrument shaft (B)
- The wrist (C)
- Tip or end effector (D)
- Instrument housing (E)

Instrument Housing (E)

The Da Vinci S, Si instruments can be differentiated by their length, housing color and graphics. The maximum total length of the shaft is 52 cm. The Da Vinci S and Si have a blue housing. Red housing is for training instrument. Light grey for Da Vinci. The S instrument are 5 cm long. The housing on the profile have two flush ports (Si) and three flush port (S). The emergency release grip is seen on the housing for release of stuck instruments. The housing also has ESU connection probe.

Once the robot is draped it is brought near the patient and attached to the laparoscopic/robotic ports. This process is called as 'docking'.

REFERENCES

1. Clayman RV, Kavoussi LR, Soper JN, et al. Laparoscopic nephrectomy: Initial case report. J Urol. 1991;146:278-82.
2. Ratner LE, Montgomery RA, Cohen C, et al. Laparoscopic live donor nephrectomy. Transplantation. 1995;60(9):1047.
3. Rané A, Rao P, Rao P. Single-port-access nephrectomy and other laparoscopic urologic procedures using a novel laparoscopic port (R-port). Urology. 2008; 72(2):260-3; discussion 263-4.
4. Gaur DD. Laparoscopic operative retroperitoneoscopy: use of a new device. J Urol. 1992;148(4):1137-9.
5. Ponsky L, Cherullo E, Moinzadeh A, et al. The Hem-o-lok clip is safe for laparoscopic nephrectomy: a multi-institutional review. Urology. 2008;71(4):593-6.
6. Mcguire J, Wright IC, Leverment JN. Surgical staplers: A review. J R Coll Surg Edinb 1997;42(1):1-9.

Energy Sources in Open, Laparoscopic and Robotic Surgery

"Heat cures when everything else fails"

—**Hippocrates**

INTRODUCTION

Surgery can be defined as the art of tissue dissection and tissue re-approximation. A variety of energy sources have been used in tissue dissection to provide energy for cutting and hemostasis. Unfortunately, many surgeons poorly understand the biophysics of these sources. For most of us, pressing the cautery pedal is like taking a leap of faith without knowing the science behind it.

Let us in the coming few pages try to understand the energy sources available in market today for different kinds of procedure.

DEFINITIONS[1]

Electrosurgery: It is the use of radiofrequency alternating current to raise the cellular temperature to vaporize or coagulate tissue.

Electrocautery is not same as electrosurgery. Electrocautery uses direct current whereas electrosurgery uses alternating current and in electrosurgery patient is a part electrical circuit.[1]

Cautery (Kauterion = hot iron): Destruction or denaturation of tissue by passive transfer of heat or application of caustic substance.

- Current = Flow of electrons during a period of time, measured in amperes
- Circuit = Pathway for the uninterrupted flow of electrons
- Voltage = Force pushing current through the resistance, measured in volts
- Impedance/Resistance = Obstacle to the flow of current, measured in ohms (impedance = resistance)

CLASSIFICATION

- Based on the type of generator used:
  - Electrosurgical
  - Further subclassified into:
    a. *Simple generator*: Monopolar/Bipolar cautery
    b. *Advanced bipolar systems*:
      1. Ligasure
      2. PK system
      3. Enseal
    c. Ultrasonic
    d. Integrated ultrasound and advance bipolar generators
    e. Argon Beam coagulator
    f. Lasers
    g. *Others*: Radio frequency, Microwave, Cryo
- Based on their use in urologic surgeries:
  - *Open surgery*: Monopolar, bipolar, vessel sealing (Ligasure, Enseal), ultrasonic, argon beam coagulator
  - *Laparoscopic surgery*: Monopolar, Bipolar, Vessel sealing (Ligasure, Enseal, PK), ultrasonic, Argon beam coagulator, laser
  - *Robotic surgery*: Monopolar, bipolar, ultrasonic, PK.

Electrosurgical Generator

Frequency spectrum (Figure 1):

A typical electrosurgical generator takes our household current of 60 cycles/second and raises the frequency to 200,000 cycles/second. Such high frequencies are radio frequencies, when current passes at such high frequency through the human body no neuromuscular stimulation occurs and patient does not get an electric shock.

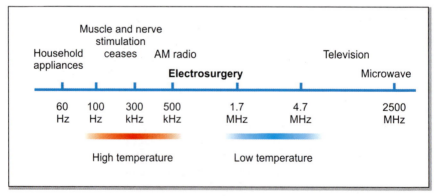

Figure 1: Frequency spectrum

Monopolar Generator[1]

They are the most commonly available electrosurgical units in all operating rooms (Figure 2).

Monopolar circuit: Generator—Active electrode—Patient—Patient return electrode.

Various waveforms generated by electrosurgical generators (Figure 3) are[1]:
- *Cut:* Waveform is constant, heat is generated rapidly leading to tissue vaporization or cutting.
- *Coagulation:* Waveform is interrupted, less heat is produced, and no tissue vaporization occurs instead coagulation occurs.
- *Blend current:* It is modification of duty cycle. Using a lower duty cycle less heat is produced and less heat produces coagulation. Conversely higher duty cycle produces lot of heat that vaporizes tissue.

ELECTROSURGICAL TISSUE EFFECTS (FIGURE 4)

Electrosurgical Cutting

By using this mode, surgeon can cut like a knife, as the intense heat produced vaporizes tissue. When the electrode is held slightly away from the tissue maximum current concentration and maximum cutting can be achieved.

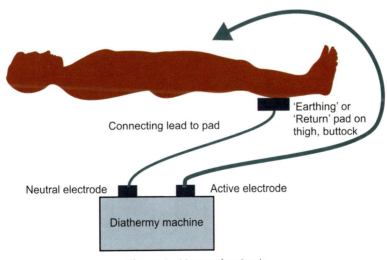

Figure 2: Monopolar circuit

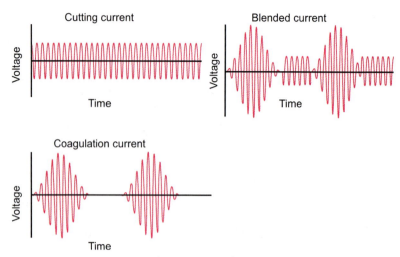

Figure 3: Waveform

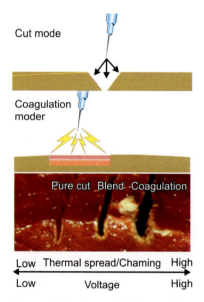

Figure 4: Electrosurgical tissue effect

Fulguration

In this mode, charring occurs involving a wider area. In fulguration mode, the duty cycle (on time) is only 6%, this leads to heating up of tissue and coagulation rather than vaporization.

Desiccation

When an electrode directly touches tissue less heat is generated as a result, the cell do not vaporize and instead dry up and form coagulum.

Surgeons can cut with coagulation current and coagulate with cutting current. Cutting current will penetrate deeper and coagulation current will have lateral spread. When coagulating with the cutting current you require less voltage and cutting with cut current also requires less voltage. The above facts have a bearing when you are using electrosurgery in laparoscopic surgery.

Bipolar[1]

In this form of electrosurgery, active and the return electrode are the part of the bipolar device and no patient plate is required. The current passes from one prong of bipolar device to the other through the tissue in between and circuit is completed (Figure 5).

ADVANCE BIPOLAR SYSTEMS

1. *Ligasure (Figure 6)*: It is advanced bipolar energy source available in surgical armamentarium today. It is combines pressure and energy to create a seal. It consists of a specialized generator system that reliably seals vessels, tissue bundles and can be used as tool for surgical ligation of tissues in open and laparoscopic surgery.

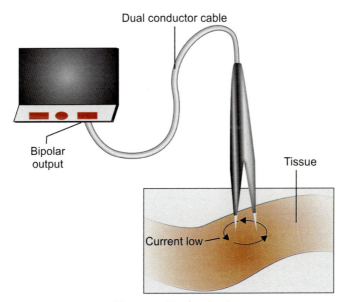

Figure 5: Bipolar circuit

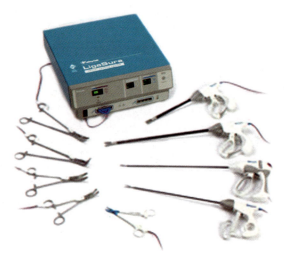

Figure 6: Ligasure

Ligasure uses higher current and lower voltage (180 V) along with optimal pressure delivery by the instruments in order to fuse the vessel walls and create a permanent seal. It has a feedback control mechanism, which gives an alarm once the tissue is adequately sealed. Vessels up to 7 mm can be reliably sealed using this device. It has minimal thermal spread and the seal site is often translucent, this allows the surgeon to look for hemostasis prior to cutting the tissue.

Sealed blood vessel can with stand a rise in blood pressure equal to three times, the systolic pressure. Sealing tissue and blood vessels with this device is as effective as suture ligation or clip application.

Ligasure devices are available for open (Ligasure precise) as well as laparoscopic surgery (Ligasure versus Ligasure lap). Ligasure is as of now not available for robotic platform.

- Reliable, consistent permanent vessel wall fusion
- Minimal thermal spread
- Reduced sticking and charring
- Seal strength than other energy-based techniques
- Seal strength comparable to existing mechanical-based techniques

2. The Gyrus PK tissue management system (Gyrus Medical, Inc, Minneapolis, Minnesota) (Figure 7): Gyrus PK system uses bipolar RF energy to seal, transect, coagulate, dissect, vaporize, resect and mobilize tissue all with the precision and control from one workstation. It is based on principle of vapor pulse coagulation (VPC). On application of the energy, tissue fluid boils producing steam which form vapor pockets, these vapor pockets coalesce to form vapor zones. This heating of the tissue causes denaturing

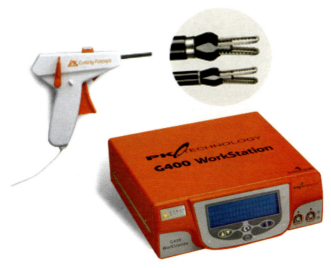

Figure 7: PK system

of vessel wall protein and coagulum formation, which occludes the vessel lumen, pulse-off periods allow tissue for cooling and moisture to return to the targeted area, greatly reducing hot spots and coagulum formation. This system provides enhanced hemostasis, uniform coagulation, minimal sticking and less thermal spread. The Gyrus PK system has its own generator, which works in tandem with its own instruments. It has application in open surgery, laparoscopy and robotic surgery. Separated instruments are developed for all types of surgery's but the generator can remain the same.

For open surgery PK, seal open forceps is available, for laparoscopy cutting forcep, dissecting forcep, hook and spatula are available. Recently the Pk dissecting forcep for robotic surgery was launched but not in common use till now.

3. Enseal™ (SurgRx, Inc. Palo Alto, CA) (Figure 8).

Ethicon Endosurgery Generator

The Enseal tissue sealing system uses an advanced bipolar technology to seal the tissue within the blades of the instrument. It uses the patented I Blade technology, which offers strong uniform compression along the tissue sealing line. Enseal uses a smart electrode technology, which includes numerous conductive particles embedded in a plate, which is temperature-sensitive. Each of these particles acts like a discrete thermostatic switch to regulate the quantity of current that passes into the tissues in contact, thereby generating heat within it. Once the tissue starts heating above a critical level, these nano-particles interrupt the flow of current and when the temperature dips below, the desired level they again reactivate the current, this cycle is continued till desired temperature is reached (temperature is regulated to a set level of 100°C.

The procedure continues until the entire tissue segment is uniformly heated and fused without charring or sticking. Less heat is needed to accomplish fusion, since the tissue volume is minimized through compression; energy is focused about the captured segment; and the vessel walls are fused through compression, protein denaturation. It can seal vessels up to 7 mm with a seal strength of 7 times the systolic pressure and has One-step actuation for both cutting and sealing. Enseal was US FDA approved in 2003.

Enseal has instruments for open surgery (e.g. super jaw tissue sealer)[2] as well as laproscopic surgery (straight and curved tissue sealer) but not for robotic arm. It has a articulating tissue sealer (G2 articulating tissue sealer)[2] which can have application in single port surgery.

Ultrasonic Generators (Figure 9)

Physics of ultrasound: Ultrasound is longitudinal wave, whose frequency is above the audible range. High power ultrasound can be harnessed to produce surgical cutting, coagulation, and dissection of tissues. This involves mechanical propagation of sound (pressure) waves from a power source via a medium to an active blade element.

Ultrasonic dissectors are of two types:

1. *Low power*: These operate at a low frequency and cleaves water containing tissues by cavitations. The organized structures with low water content are sparse, e.g. arteries, bile ducts, etc. For example, (ultrasonic cavitational aspirators) bring liver surgery and neurosurgery (Cusa, Selector). They do not achieve coagulation.
2. *High power*: These systems operate at high frequency of 55.5 KHz, which cleave loose areolar tissues by frictional heating and, therefore, cut and coagulate the edges simultaneously. In laparoscopic surgery, high power ultrasonic systems are utilized extensively. Ultrasurgical devices consists of a generator, handpiece, and blade. The ultrasonic transducer is housed

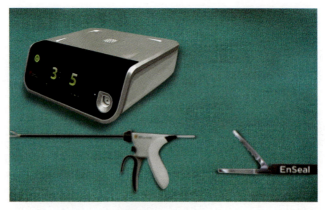

Figure 8: Enseal

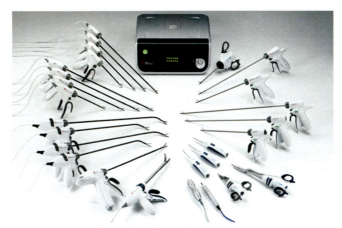

Figure 9: Ultrasonic generator

in the handpiece, a collection of piezoelectric crystals sandwiched under pressure between metal cylinders. The transducer is attached to a mount, which is then connected to the blade extender and blade. The harmonic scalpel cools the handpiece with air. AutoSonix and Sonosurg systems have a large diameter handpiece made of heat dissipating materials to remove the heat and stop heat build up.

Once activated the electrical energy is passed to handpiece, piezoelectric ceramic disks in hand piece become excited, this electrical energy is transferred into mechanical energy. Mechanical energy is amplified at nodes in shaft of the instrument and reaches a maximum amplitude of 55,500 cycle/sec at blade tip, when in contact with tissue pressure causes coaptation of vessels, H+ bonds are broken and cell protein is denatured forming sticky coagulum.

Ultrasonic hook or spatula blade can coagulate blood vessels within the 2 mm diameter range quite easily and also the scissors can coagulate vessels up to 5 mm in diameter. Heat generated using the harmonic is limited to temperature below 80°C. This leads to reduced tissue charring and desiccation and also minimizes the zone of thermal injury. Ultrasonic surgery causes slower coagulation than that observed with either electrosurgery or laser surgery, but is as effective.

Incisions made with the ultrasonically activated scalped or cold steel scalpel heal almost identically and, therefore, are superior to electrosurgically made incisions.

Due to the vibration from the active blade, the coagulated tissue does not stick to the active element, this is a unique feature of ultrasonic coagulator as compared to other sources. Also there is less charring compared to other sources, leading to better visualization of the tissue planes thereby improving the surgical precision. It also has a second cutting mechanism, which is the particular "power cutting" offered by a relatively sharp blade vibrating 55,500 times per second over a distance of 80 μm. Excessive heating of ultrasonic dissectors causing collateral damage is well documented in clinical practice, therefore, one must be careful while using this instrument as a dissector. Ultrasonic surgical dissection allows coagulation and cutting with less instrument exchanges (reduction in operating time), decreased smoke and no current.

Ultrasonic dissectors are available for both open (harmonic focus) and laparoscopic surgery (Harmonic ACE).

Now Harmonic ACE™ curved shears is available for da Vinci S/si system.

Salient features
- Mechanical energy at 55,500 vibrations/sec
- Disrupts hydrogen bonds and forms a coagulum
- Temperature by Harmonic Scalpel—80°C
- Temperature through electrocoagulation—200–300°C
- Minimal collateral damage
- Multifunctional instruments
- Less tissue sticking
- Less smoke formation
- No stray energy
- No neuromuscular stimulation
- No electrical energy to or through the patient

Factors affecting cutting and coagulation in ultrasonic devices
- Tissue tension
- Blade sharpness
- Time
- Power level
- Grip force
  It can be sterilized by autoclaving/ETO/Strerrad.

Integrated Ultrasound and Advanced Bipolar Generators

The Thunderbeat™ (Olympus), was the first device to integrate the ultrasonic and advanced bipolar generator. Both the generators can be used interchangeably. Ethicon has also come up with an integrated generator ETHICON ENDO-SURGERY™ compatible with all harmonic and enseal devices. The sealing capabilities of this device is necessarily same as ultrasonic or advanced bipolar depending on the generator used.

Comparison of Various Energy Sources

Device	Safety: Minimal thermal spread	Vessel sealing Efficacy on vessels ≤7 mm	Efficiency: Treatment time	Consistency: Independent of user	Utility: Multiple uses
Harmonic scalpel	1 mm	Poor	Excellent	Poor	Excellent
Gyrus PK	2–6 mm	Poor	Excellent	Fair	Fair
LigaSure V	2–3 mm	Excellent	Good	Excellent	Fair
EnSeal	1 mm	Excellent	Poor	Excellent	Poor

Argon Beam Coagulator[1]

The argon beam coagulator (ABC) uses radiofrequency electrical energy, which is delivered to tissue through a jet of argon gas. It provides noncontact, monopolar, electrothermal hemostasis. Argon is inert, noncombustible. Easily ionizes, making it more conductive and safe medium for electric current to pass. The dept of penetration is less and less smoke is produced.

It is particularly useful in repair of solid organ injury and finds its utility in cases of partial nephrectomy in urological spectrum of surgeries. Drawback of argon beam coagulators in laparoscopy is that it increases the intra-abdominal pressures dangerously and may cause fatal gas embolism (Figure 10).

Properties of Argon

- Inert
- Noncombustible
- Easily ionized by RF energy
- Creates bridge between electrode and the tissue
- Displaces nitrogen and oxygen
- Advantages of argon beam coagulator
- Decrease smoke and odor
- Decreases blood loss, rebleeding and tissue damage
- Flexible

LASERS (Light amplification through stimulated emission of radiation): All the discussion about lasers in urology revolves around prostatectomy's. Lasers have been used in laparoscopy. Lasers described for laparoscopic use have

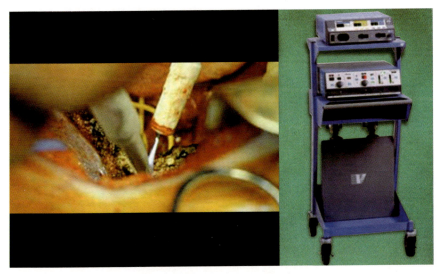

Figure 10: Argon beam coagulator

been CO_2, diode, KTP, holmium, thulium. Though the use is still not wide spread there have been many animal studies and few clinical trials. CO_2 laser has been used in open surgeries like wide local excision for carcinoma penis, head and neck surgeons used it for excision of head and neck malignancies.

In laparoscopy CO_2 laser has been used in gynecological practice to treat endometriosis, etc.

Lot of experimental work in animal models has been done demonstrating utility of laser in laparoscopic partial nephrectomy. Clinical studies have also demonstrated use of thulium and holmium lasers for laparoscopic partial nephrectomy.

A study by KUN Pang et al demonstrated use for thulium laser for resection of distal ureter with bladder cuff in case of TCC kidney. An Italian study has demonstrated use of thulium laser for partial nephrectomy. On the whole use of lasers in laparoscopic surgeries is yet to find its distinct place but as the search for a better cutting and coagulating energy source continues more studies on lasers in laparoscopy are going to tell us if lasers in laparoscopy are here to stay. **Note:** Details about Physics of laser can be found elsewhere in the book.

Radiofrequency Ablation

It consists of a probe, which may be a simple needle, or in form of prongs. The probe is mounted on a radiofrequency generator. The generator sends radiofrequency waves through the needle, RF energy causes atoms in the cells to vibrate that will create friction. This generates heat (as much as 100°C) and leads to coagulative necrosis. The use of radiofrequency ablation as energy source is limited.

Gill et al have studied animal models of laparoscopic and percutaneous radiofrequency ablation of part of kidney. The application of RF ablation is more studied in malignancy, e.g. ablation of small renal masses and carcinoma prostate. It is as of now less likely to be used as a hemostatic agent.

Microwave Ablation

Like radiofrequency ablation microwave ablation is also being used for tumor ablation rather than as a hemostatic agent for surgery. It is an alternate way of producing thermal coagulation of tissue, microwaves induce ultrahigh speed (2450 MHz) alternating field current, resulting in rotation of water molecule. This heats up the tissue causing coagulative necrosis. Majority of experience comes from its use in hepatocellular carcinoma. It is being used in management of small renal masses and carcinoma prostate. It can be used laparoscopically as well as image guided.

Cryotherapy

The cell destruction by rapidly cooling the cell and the thawing is the principle of cryotherapy. It can be used laparoscopically as well as under image guidance. It is being used in management of small renal masses and carcinoma prostate. As of now it cannot be used for cutting and coagulating tissue in open and minimal access surgery.

SAFETY CONSIDERATION[1]

- *Patient pad placement*: Patient plate should be in contact over a large surface area at least 100 square cm. One should avoid bony prominences; Soft pads are better than metallic plates as they give uniform area of contact. The pads should be placed near the area of interest.
- *Demodulated current*: Modern generators filter demodulated current so that only electrical current of 250 – 2000 kHz is delivered. Demodulated currents occur in common practice when an active electrode is activated off metal after which touched towards the metal, like the common practice of 'buzzing a hemostat'. Demodulated currents produces neuromuscular activity. The flickering movements in laparoscopic surgery may be caused by demodulation of current to diaphragm and adjoining muscles.
- During minimally invasive surgery[1]:
  - *Direct application*: Direct application of active electrode to an unintended area causes tissue injury.
  - *Direct coupling*: When the activated active electrode touches a nearby metallic instrument it energizes it and this stray energy may find its way to the patient plate causing injury. Like if a monopolar hook touches a laparoscopic telescope, if the telescope is in turn in contact with bowel. The energized telescope will cause thermal injury to the bowel (Figure 11).
  - *Insulation failure*: Breaks in the insulation can cause energy to stray and cause tissue injury. For example, if a portion of monopolar hook has an insulation break and this area comes in contact with bowel it will cause the current to leak and may lead to bowel injury (Figure 12).
  - *Capacitative coupling*: Capacitance is the charge generated when an insulator separates two conductors. This charge has a tendency to complete circuit and cause surrounding organ injury. For example, Hybrid cannula with suction and hook have a metallic hook covered by a insulator which is fixed within a metallic suction cannula. The insulator between to metallic conductor acts as a capacitor and when it comes in contact with adjacent bowel the stray energy may be leaked causing a bowel injury (Figure 13).

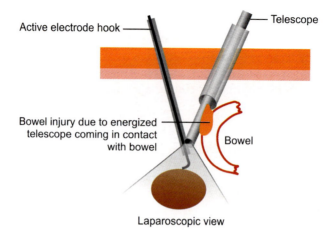

Figure 11: Direct coupling of current

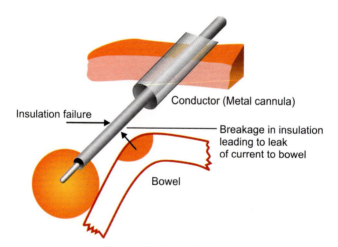

Figure 12: Insulation failure

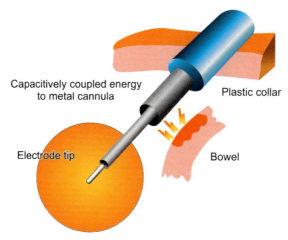

Figure 13: Capacitative coupling

REFERENCES

1. *www.asit.org/assets/documents/Prinicpals_in_electrosurgery.pdf*
2. *http://www.ethicon.com/healthcare-professionals/products/advanced-energy/enseal/enseal-g2-tissue-sealers*
3. *http://medical.olympusamerica.com/products/thunderbeat-1*

Accessories

URETERIC CATHETER

Material

The material is polyethylene with radiopaque coating, a Luer lock/simple adaptor is provided at proximal end of the catheter for attaching the syringe. Markings—Single marking at every centimeter. The marking is as follows:

- 5 cm—single mark
- 10 cm—two marks
- 15 cm—3 marks
- 20 cm—4 marks
- 25–5 marks
- 30—one bold mark
- 35–2 marks
- 40–3 marks
- 45–4 marks
- 50–5 marks

No marking beyond 50 cm. The length generally is 70 cm.

Types of Ureteric Catheter

The ureteric catheters are classified depending on the tip configuration:

1. *Open end catheter (Figures 1A and C)*[1]: Single opening at the tip, no side openings. It is used for drainage and performing pyelography. It can be passed over glidewire across obstruction or kink.

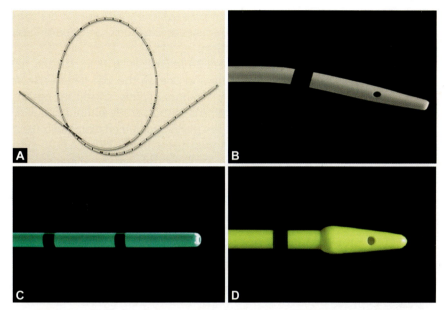

Figures 1A to D: (A) Ureteric catheter with markings; (B) Angle tipped urereric catheter; (C) Open end ureteric catheter; (D) Cone tipped ureteric catheter

2. *Close end catheter*[2]: This always comes with a stylet. It has a round blunt tip and two holes on the side.
3. *Cone tipped ureteric catheter*[3] *(Figure 1D)*: Available in different sizes. The size is described as the size of tip and the catheter. The tip is pointed and a hole just proximal to the tip. This is used for bulb ureterogram. Generally, available as 5 Fr and 14 Fr (bulb) and 4 Fr and 8 Fr (bulb)(cook). This has to be back loaded if it is 14 Fr, smaller bulb can be passed without back loading through a larger cystoscope sheath.
4. *Angled tip ureteral catheter (Coude)*[4] *(Figure 1B)*: This was used for negotiating an awkward ureteric orifice and kinks in the ureter. With the guidewire in use these have become obsolete. They can be angled at either 20° or 40°.
5. *Whistle tip catheter*[5]: It is oblique (like a whistle) open end catheter. It is used for performing a retrograde ureterogram.
6. *Balloon ureteric catheter:* It has a separate channel where the balloon can be inflated.
7. *Pig tail ureteric catheter*[6]: Available as 70 cm and 90 cm. It has a single curl at the kidney end. This can be kept as self-retaining ureteric catheter.

8. *Echotip open-end ureteral catheter*[7] *(Figure 2A and B)*: Used for drainage and irrigation. The Echotip® band enhances ultrasonic and fluoroscopic visualization of the catheter tip location.
9. *Double lumen ureteric catheter (Figures 3A to C)*: It is 10 Fr in size and has two channels one opening at the tip and one on the side (Figures 3A to C). The openings are approximately 1 cm apart. This is used for passing additional safety catheter or performing a contrast study without removing the preplaced wire. It is 50 cm long. The placement lumen diameter is 0.038 inch (0.97 mm), while the injection lumen diameter is 0.050 inch (1.26 mm). A variant in the form of flexitip is also available. This catheter eliminates the need for multiple catheterization. The flexitip is intended for a traumatic catheterization into the ureter (adapted from Cook catalog supplement, 1996).

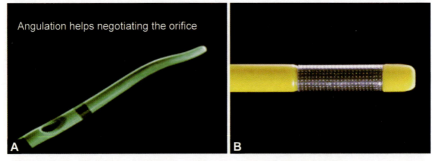

Angulation helps negotiating the orifice

Figures 2A and B: (A) Angled tipped ureteral catheter; (B) Echo tipped ureteral catheter

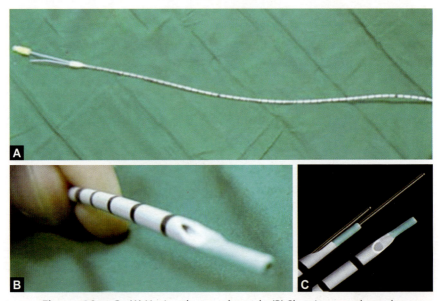

Figures 3A to C: (A) Hosing the two channels; (B) Showing two channels; (C) Showing two guidewires

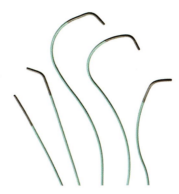

Figure 3D: Torqueable tip ureteral access catheter

10. *Spiral tip ureteral access catheter*[8]: Used for drainage and retrograde pyelogram. The spiral tip aids in negotiation of a tortuous or partially obstructed ureter. The large side port below the spiral allows passage of a guidewire.
11. *Torqueable tip ureteral access*: Catheter used for negotiation of a tortuous or partially obstructed ureter (Figure 3D).

Guidewires

They are used for access or dilatation of tract. There are different types of guide-wire straight tip, flexible tip, stiff, hydrophilic, etc.
Guidewires can be classified by the following properties:
1. *Size*: Size—0.018–0.038 inches, length usually—150 cm
2. Tip design
    – Straight tip
    – Angled tips negotiate awkward located ureteral orifices (i.e. in median lobe hypertrophy)
    – J tips are beneficial in preventing ureteral perforation, because the leading edge of the wire is an 'elbow,' which is less traumatic than the relatively sharper end of a straight wire. They are especially useful in patients who have impacted ureteral calculi or ureteral tortuosity. It is also useful in PCNL.
3. Surface coating—Characteristics (Figures 4A and B)
    – Most standard *stainless steel* guidewires are coated with polytetrafluo-roethylene (PTFE).
    – Hydrophilic-coated wire–Glidewire. Its *superelastic nitinol alloy* core tapers gradually at the tip and is covered in polyurethane with a thin hydrophilic coating.
* *Shaft rigidity*: *Three main parts of guidewire*: A spring guide, an inner core wire, and a mandrel.
    Typically, the spring guide is a round wire tightly wrapped around the inner metal core and mandrel. The core provides strength and stability to the wire, whereas the spring guide acts as a track for the smooth passage of instruments.

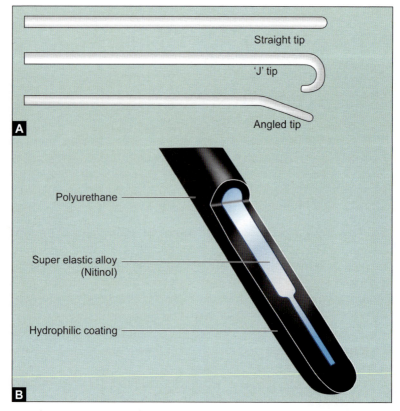

Figures 4A and B: (A) Types of guidewire; (b) Parts of guidewire

The inner core is usually welded to the spring guide (fixed core); however, some wires have nonfixed (movable) cores. The tip can be flexible for 8 cm.

Types

1. *Stainless steel core guidewire (fix core)*: Stainless steel core with PTFE coating. It is used for dilatation of tract or stent placement
   - Advantage—more stable and does not slip out
   - Disadvantage—more prone to get kinked and outer coating may come out if there is a kink, high chances of perforation (ureteric) or submucosal passage.
2. Nitinol core hydrophilic guidewire—(Glidewire)[9]
   - Core—nitinol core for flexibility
   - Coating—polyurethane coating for smooth soft surface has tungsten added for radiopacity
   - Hydrophilic material—(M polymer) which causes water to stick on surface to make it smooth and slippery

- Advantage
    - smooth and atraumatic so used to pass across stones, stricture, kinks, etc.
    - smooth coating so wire does not kink
- Disadvantage
    - very slippery can come out easily.
- Diameters (Inch)—0.018, 0.025, 0.035 and 0.038
- Lengths—80 cm, 150 cm, 180 cm and 260 cm
3. *Amplatz fixed core guidewire (Boston scientific)*: This is a superstiff guidewire[10]—Stainless steel core with PTFE coating, more stiff wire.
Used for PCNL tract dilatation, ureteral sheath or stent placement.
Can be stiff, extrastiff or ultrastiff. Extrastiffness is given by the larger flat mandrel.
4. *Zebra guidewire[11]*: Nitinol core with smooth PTFE coating with blue and white stripes, lubricious (Uro-Glide)™ coating. Platinum distal tip for better fluoroscopic visualization. It had advantages of both guidewire and glidewire and disadvantage of none. It has advantage of a radioopaque tip, so tip is like a glidewire and shaft like a guidewire. It is Kink resistant, better handling qualities and flexible tip.
5. *Sensor wire (Boston scientific) (Hybrid wire)*: Nitinol core, distal 5 cm has hydrophilic coating, it has a floppy tip, flat wire outer core, rest of the wire has a smooth PTFE coating. It has tungsten filled radiopaque tip for fluoroscopic visualization.
6. *Road runner wire (cook medical)*: It has nitinol core, platinum tip, hydrophilic polymer coating. It is available as standard shaft or stiff shaft.
7. *Biwire—double floppy tip[12]*: Flexible tips at both ends. Hydrophilic coating with nitinol core. One flexible tip used to pass atraumatically in ureter and other flexible tip causes less damage to endoscopes on rail loading it over wire.

Double J Stent (Figure 5A)

Double J (DJ) stent can be classified on basis of:
1. Length.
2. Size.
3. Material.
4. Miscellaneous.
1. *Classification on basis of length*: Length of stent is the straight part of stent and not from tip to tip.
For tortuous ureter larger length is necessary. Generally length are variable between 12 cm and 30 cm.
Different ways to measure length of DJ are:
a. Formula for deciding the length of the stent
    - *Pediatric age group*: Age +10 (in cm)
    - *Adults*: Height from 149.5 cm to 178.5 cm—DJ length of 22–26 cm

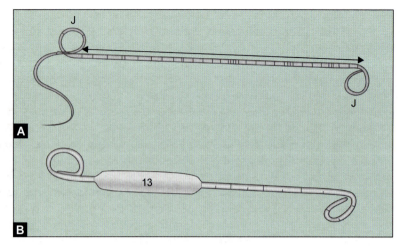

Figures 5A and B: Double J Stents: (A) The length of the stent is measured excluded the "J"; (B) Endopyelotomy stent

b. On plain X-ray KUB (of actual size) length of DJ required is equal to length measured from xiphisternum to pubic symphysis.
c. In an IVP plate (of actual size) length of the DJ required is equal to distance between VUJ and PUJ.
2. *Classification on basis of size*: Size is measured at the shaft and represents at the outer diameter of stent. It generally varies from 3 Fr to 8 Fr.
3. Classification on basis of material used.
1. Polymers:
    – Polyurethane
    – Silicone
    – C Flex – (Cook urological)
    – Sof- flex (Cook urological)
    – Percuflex (Boston Scientific)
2. Metallic (Resonance, memocath)
3. Biodegradable.

Types of Stents

A. *Polyurethane stents*[13]: It has good tensile strength and can be passed over guidewire and does not collapse on extrinsic pressure easily. Rigidity causes more stent related discomfort and can damage ureter. More prone to encrustation and colonization, should not be left for more than 6 months ideally should be removed within 3 months.
B. *Silicone stent*: It has high biodurability and biocompatibility but it has poor tensile strength and susceptible for extrinsic compression. Poor strength requires low inner diameter to outer diameter ratio which leads to smaller lumen. It has poor drainage efficiency as compared to polyurethane. The poor coil retention leads to spontaneous migration.

C. *Percuflex, C-flex, Sof flex*[14]: These are made of proprietary copolymers softer and less bladder irritation. More biocompatible and can be left for longer time. These have higher inner diameter/outer diameter ratio and hence have bigger lumen. This property is permitted by these copolymers with higher strengths. These stents have hydrophilic polymer coating for smooth surface and easy insertion.[15]

D. *Metallic stent (Resonance stent)(Cook medical)*[16]: It is made of special metallic material, unlike other stent it is not hollow and is solid cylindrical stent. Preferably used for extrinsic compression of ureter. Resistant to encrustation can be left for 12 months.

E. *Memocath—Nitinol (Nickel/titanium alloy[17])*: It expands to predetermined size at warm temperature 65°C. Resistant to encrustation and can be left for longer duration, used for variable length of strictures, benign and malignant.

Steps of Memocath Deployment

- Measure the stricture and mark it on skin with radiopaque markers
- Park a guide wire across
- Use access sheath with dilator to go beyond the stricture
- Remove the dilator
- Pass memocath deployment system from within the access sheath
- Withdraw the sheath below the stricture
- After ensuring the appropriate level of stent, put sterile NS (normal saline) at 65°C
- Stent expands and is held in place by expanded cranial end.
- Unscrew the rest of the assembly and remove the sheath.

A. *Drug-eluting stents*: They are coated with varying chemicals to decrease encrustation or biofilm formation. Still under trial.
  - Heparin—provides antiadhesive surface which resists encrustation and biofilm formation
  - Hydrogel coated, PTFE coated, antimicrobial triclosan, antibody coated, Phospholipid polymer coated, titanium nitric oxide coated.

B. *Biodegradable/Bioabsorbable stent*: Polyglycolide, Poly D, L lactide, Poly L lactide and Uriprene are biodegradable polymeric. Complete stent absorption occurs over a varied period. Data are inadequate for human use. Stent polymers are not radiopaque and the radiopacity is afforded by metallic salts of barium or bismuth. Stents are available with more than one coil at end which may make its use possible as multilength stent.

Miscellaneous Stents

A. *Dangler stents*[18] are usual DJ with additional nylon or prolene wire loops dangling out of the stent end. This helps in its removal without cystoscopy.

B. *Endopyelotomy stent (Figure 5B)*[19–21]: Used after endopyelotomy or endourological management of upper ureteric stricture or PUJ obstruction, to maintain the lumen of the upper ureter and PUJ. Proximal end is wide with narrow distal end like usual stent.

Tubes and Urethral Catheters

A urinary catheter is a tube placed in the body to collect urine from the bladder. Urinary catheters are available in variety of sizes (8 Fr–26 Fr), materials (latex, silicone, Teflon™), and types (Foley, straight, coude tip). Size is usually measured in French catheter scale or 'French units' (Fr) or Charriere (Ch) which measures the outside diameter of catheters (1 Fr is equivalent to 0.33 mm, or 1/77" of diameter).

French also indicates the circumference in millimeter, i.e. 16 Fr catheter has 16 mm circumference (Circumference = π d = 3.14 × diameter = 3 × diameter).

Catheters can be classified as:[22]
1. Single-use (Nonindwelling).
2. Indwelling (Foley) catheters.

Types of Urethral Catheters

Depending on retention mechanism
1. Simple catheter (Nonindwelling):
    – Simple rubber catheter (K90 = 14 Fr, K91 = 10 Fr, Teiman, female catheter, Nelaton catheter). K90, K91 are now available as R90 and R91.
    – Metallic catheters, etc.
2. Self-retaining catheters:
    – Foley catheter
    – Gibbons catheter
    – Malecots catheter
    – Pig tail catheter.

Description of Individual Catheters

Red Rubber Catheter (Robinson Catheter)

Made up of India rubber for single use to empty bladder, it has two eyelet (two opposing eyes) which provide high flow of urine. It is radiopaque due to lead oxide content.[23] Available in 8–22 Fr size.[24] Red rubber catheter used is declining as India rubber is irritant to urothelium.

Nelaton Catheter

Nelaton catheter is a simple tube with one hole at side (rounded tip ensure an easier insertion) or at tip ('open-ended' catheter), and a connecting piece at the opposite end to connect to a collecting bag. Most are made up of PVC (polyvinylchloride) and have some rigidity and radiopacity.

Foley Catheters

Foley catheter is a self-retaining catheter because of balloon mechanism at the end, balloon connected to a nozzle with a valve mechanism to the other end through a small tube running through the wall of catheter. Balloon capacity is mentioned on the side of nozzle end.[25] Apart from the 'all known' Foley catheter the other contributions that Foley is credited with are:

1. Foleys completely rotatable resectoscope.
2. A hydraulic cystolithotomy table.
3. Pressurized fluid delivery system.
4. A Canister which would inflate any balloon catheter.
5. A urethral sphincter device.

Types of Foley catheters (based on type of material used):

1. Simple latex Foley catheter.
2. Siliconized latex Foley catheters (Silicolatex).
3. Silicone Foley catheters.

Types Based on Use

1. Simple Foley catheter
2. Three-way hemostatic catheters
3. Hematuria catheters.

Different Types of end Holes and Catheter Tips

These are the types of catheter tips:

1. *Straight tip*: This is the most common type.
2. *The Delinotte tip (also called Mercier tip/Coude tip)*: It is same as straight tip but with bent end for easy passage through prostate.
3. *The Couvelaire tip* (also called the whistle tip): Helps in easy passage of debris, clots from the bladder.
4. Dufour tip (combination of coude and whistle tip).
5. *The Tiemann tip*: Rigid slightly bent tip and bulbous end for easy passage through prostate.

Siliconized Latex Foley Catheters

Have a silicon coating over latex, latex is supposed to be irritant to the urothelium of the urinary tract leading to microulcerations and stricture. Some patients have allergy to latex too. To overcome above drawbacks silicon coating was done over latex as former is considered to be urothelium friendly. With time silicone layer may be damaged exposing underlying latex, restricting their use for 2–3 weeks only, needing removal or replacement after that.

Silicone Foley catheters: Completely made of silicone and are costlier compared to siliconized latex catheter. These catheters are often transparent but they also come in white, blue, green and other colors. Main advantage is that they are less irritant, resistant to wear and tear, less prone to encrustation and are more rigid than siliconized latex catheters (easy passage in obstructive prostate gland).

The balloon when empty forms a slight thickening leading to slight increase in external diameter by French or two which may sometimes make passage difficult through stricture. Because of inert nature they can be placed in bladder for 6–8 weeks.

Three-way Hemostatic Catheters

Also called as three way catheters, they are specialized Foley catheters, have an extra nozzle at the end connected to an extra tube in the wall of the catheter that opens distally to the balloon used for continuous irrigation. These catheters are often of a larger diameter (20–24 Fr) which allows large debris to pass through the catheter. Catheter is reinforced with steel or nylon spiral meshed inside the tube wall or some type of catheter are made up of more rigid type of material, to prevent collapse when suction is applied for removal of debris. Tip has a wide hole for removal of debris.

Various Size Parameters and Color Coding of Catheters (Table 1 and Figure 6)

Each catheter has a color code at connecting piece or the filling opening of the balloon in Foley type catheter which denotes the external diameter of the catheter.

3-Way Foley Hematuria Catheters[26] (Figure 7)

Large eyeholes in the hematuria catheters reduce the risk of clots blocking the eye and funnel strength is maximized to resist collapse during aspiration of clots.

Tiemann Catheter (Figure 8)

Tip is bulbous, coude and relatively rigid because of the gentle curve it is easy to pass through the urethra. Color code is same as Foleys.

Nephrostomy Tubes (Figures 9A and B)

The nephrostomy tube helps to drain the kidney after the procedure, acts as a conduit to remove residual stones after a PCNL if they are detected on a post-operative film; in addition the nephrostomy tubes also help to tamponade any bleeding.

TABLE 1: Color coding for foley catheter

Channel size	Balloon size	Color	Length (cm)
8 Fr	3 cc	Aquamarine	30
10 Fr	3 cc	Black	30
12 Fr	5–10 cc	White	40
14 Fr	5–10 cc	Green	40
16 Fr	5–10 cc	Orange	40
18 Fr	5–10 cc	Red	40
20 Fr	10–20 cc	Yellow	40
22 Fr	10–20 cc	Purple	40
24 Fr	10–20 cc	Blue	40

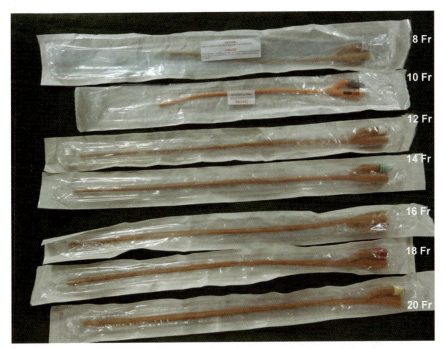

Figure 6: Various bi-way Foley catheters with color coding

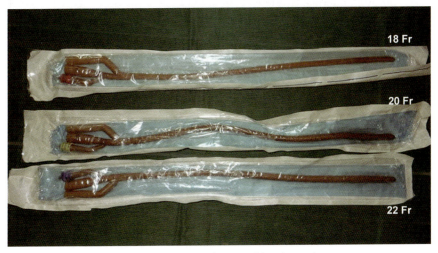

Figure 7: Triway catheters with color codes

The varieties of nephrostomy tubes available are:
1. *Councilman catheter*: This is a modified Foleys catheter, with a end on hole. This type of nephrostomy drainage is useful if the nephrostomy tube requires frequent changes.

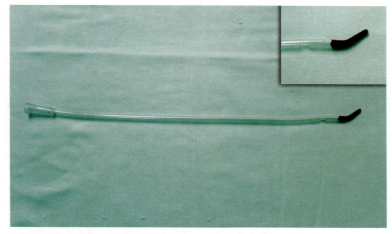

Figure 8: Tieman catheter with characteristic distal end and proximal tip

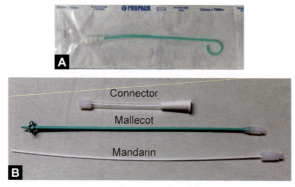

Figures 9A and B: (A) Pig tail catheter; (B) Mallecots continous drainage catheter with mandarin and connector

2. *Kaye's Tamponade balloon*: Originally the catheter was designed to arrest post-PCNL bleeding. The tamponade is provided by the balloon and the central channel provides drainage.
3. *Nelaton catheter (Figure 10A)*: The catheters range in size from 12 Fr to 28 Fr. This is the preferred method of drainage after PCNL.
4. *Foley catheters*: These are used for long term drainage and in those patients which require repeat tube changes. Disadvantage is, it is not radiopaque.
5. *Mallecots catheter (Figure 9B)*: These catheters have a flower at the end of catheter as self-retaining mechanism which open when 'mandarin' a sort of stick inside the lumen of catheter is removed. "Mandarin" keeps the tip flat during insertion and removal. These catheters are less secure then Foley as they tend to fall out with firm pull. Not widely used as urethral catheters, mainly used as nephrostomy catheter.
6. Depezzers catheters

7. Re-entry catheters (Figures 10B and C)
8. Circle nephrostomy tubes.

Baskets and Retropulsion Devices (Figure 11)

1. N Circle™ basket[27] (Cook medical, Spencer, IN)—*Peculiarities*
   It is a tipless manipulator for stone removal. It made up of nitinol sizes, 1.5, 2.2, 3.0 and 4.5 Fr.
   The length available is 65 cm (flexible nephroscope) and 115 (flexible URS). It does not occupy much space and hence can be opened in small calyx. Once the basket is opened the diameter is either 2 cm or 1 cm in size.
2. Ncompass™ basket[28] (cook Medical, Spencer, IN)—*Peculiarities*
   Multiwire geometry, made of nitinol, tipless, available in two sizes, 1.7 Fr, 2.4 Fr, length 115 cm, basket diameter after opening—1 and 1.5 cm. It does not occupy much space and hence can be opened in small calyx. It has 12–16 tightly weaned wires for intact removal of multiple fragments.
3. Ngage™ basket[28] (Cook Medical, Spencer, IN)—*Peculiarities*
   Stone extractor (ureter or calyx), engages, reposition and releases the stone as required. Available as 1.7 and 2.2 Fr and 115 cm in length, open diameter is 8 or 11mm. The basket configuration on opening is triangular in shape.
4. Nforce™[29](Cook Medical, Spencer, IN)
   Nitinol helical stone extractor (nitinol helical stone extractor)
5. Graspit™ (Boston scientific)[30]
6. Captura™ helical stone extractor (Cook medicals)[31] Sheath 1.7–4.5 Fr, a similar basket from Boston scientific is called as Gemini™ helical stone extractor.[31,32]
7. Segura hemisphere stone retrieval basket[33] (Boston scientific, Natick, MA).

Peculiarities

1. Zero tip nontraumatic. Nitinol
2. Working length, 120 or 90 cm

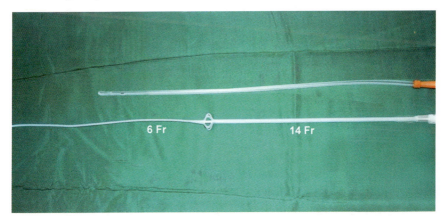

Figures 10A to C: (A) Nelaton catheter; (B) and (C) Reentry catheter

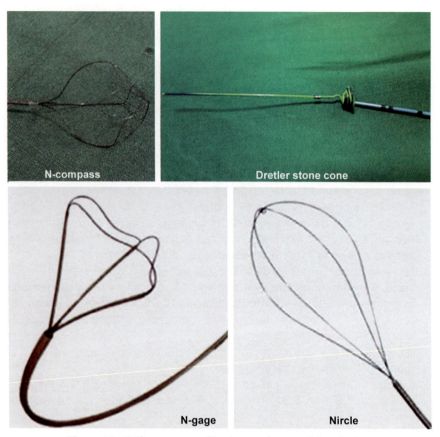

Figure 11: Different types of baskets and retropulsion devices

3. Sheath size, 2.4, 3.0 or 4.5 Fr
4. Basket diameter is 16 or 20 mm
5. Sheath material of polyimide or PTFE
6. They are available as 4, 3 and 6 wire basket.

Two Types

a. *Round wire*: To prevent ureteral trauma, they have 4 wire configured.
b. *Flat wire*: Maintain basket configuration even during difficult stone manipulation. They are 3 or 6 wire configured (Boston scientific catalogue).

Retropulsion Devices

These devices are used for preventing retropulsion of stone into the pelvicalyceal system:

1. NTrap basket[34] (Cook Medical, Spencer, IN)
   – It is used as a antireteropulsion device.
   – Basket configuration (7 mm umbrella configuration on opening).
   – It is 2.8 Fr and 145 cm.

2. Stone Cone[35] (Boston Scientific, Natick MA)
   Made of Nitinol and is available as either 7 mm or 10 mm coil with 3 Fr shaft made of PTFE
3. CoAx Stone Control Device[36] (Accordion Medical)
   Made of polyurethane film which conforms to the shape of the ureter and prevents migration.
4. Backstop[37] (Boston Scientific)
   It is a thermo sensitive polymer that is water soluble. It is deployed with access sheath like device and, thereafter, washed away with cold saline. (**See Table 2** for specifications).

Urethral Balloon Dilators

The urethral balloon dilators are used to dilate the male and female urethra to treat stricture disease. They are intended for one time use. They are 29 cm long and can be available with or without coude tip. They are available either as 9.0 Fr or 7.0 Fr in size. The inflated balloon diameter is 8.7 mm in either sizes. The balloon length is 18 cm. The balloon can withstand 6 atm pressure (90 psi). They are intended for one time use. A 0.038 inch wire can pass through its lumen.

URETERIC DILATOR

Ureteral dilators are: active and passive.

TABLE 2: Sizes/length and other specifications for baskets and retropulsion devices

Model	Available size (Fr)	Available basket size (mm)	Length (cm)	Features
Dimension (Bard)	2.4, 3.0	10, 13, 16	115	Articulating four wire, zero tip
Expand 212 (Bard)	3.0	11	90, 115	Articulating, 2-1-2-1, wire design filiform tip
Escape (Boston scientific)	1.9	11, 15	90, 120	4 wire cage with channel for 200 micron laser fiber
Optiflex (Boston scientific)	1.3	6, 7, 9, 11	90, 120	Rotates 360°, can entrap small fragments with preservation of vision
Zerotip (Boston scientific)	1.9, 2.4, 3.0	12, 16	90, 120	Zero tip helps entrapment near parenchyma
N Circle (Cook Medical)	2.4	10, 20	115	Triangular shape allows very large wire mass, tipless mass
NForce (Cook medical)	2.2, 3.2		115	3 wire
NGage (Cook Medical)	1.7, 2.2	8, 11	115	Allows repositioning

PASSIVE DILATORS: DJ STENTS

Active Dilators

1. *Single step (Figure 12A)*: Long Tapered Ureteral Dilator (Nottingham) –6/12 Fr or 6/14 Fr, tip is 6 Fr and gradually diameter increases to 12 or 14 Fr, it is made of polyethylene and is 60 cm long. Ureter can be dilated by single passage.
2. *Serial teflon ureteral dilator (Figure 12B)*: 6, 8, 9, 10, 11, 12, 14, 16, 18 Fr, they have to be passed one after the other to dilate the ureter.
3. *Ureteral balloon dilator (Figure 12C)*: It is around 65 cm in length and balloon is 4–5 mm in width on inflation and 4–6 cm in length. In collapsed state it is 3–7 Fr depending on make. Available as Passport, Ascend, etc.

Access Sheath

Flexible ureterorenoscopy can be performed with or without an access sheath. Ureteral access sheath facilitates multiple passes into ureter, reduces operative time, minimize patient morbidity, and improves overall outcome of the procedure. It maintains low intrapelvic pressure (<20 cm water with pressurized irrigation up to 200 cm water) by allowing return of irrigant fluid through the sheath and around the ureteroscope (Table 3). Thus, if repeated passes of FURS or prolonged surgery is expected, then an access sheath is placed. Ureteral access sheaths are inserted over a super-stiff working guidewire, either directly or after serial ureteric dilatation using ureteric balloon dilator or serial dilators. Among the available access sheaths, the Cook Flexor (Figures 13A and B) sheath has been found to be more resistant to both buckling at the ureteral orifice and kinking after removal of the inner dilator.[4]

Parts

Access sheaths have an inner dilator and outer sheath. The dilator has a pointed conical tip with a channel for passage over guidewire. The proximal end of the dilator has a clipping mechanism to fix the dilator to the sheath. The sheath is cylindrical with a widened flange at the proximal end. The tip of the sheath has a circular radiopaque marker. The sheath is coated with a microthin layer of hydrophilic polymer to create a low friction surface. In dual channel access sheaths (e.g. Cook Flexor DL with 3 Fr secondary channel), there is a secondary channel for passage of guidewire, basket or laser fiber (Figures 13A and B).

Available Sizes

Access sheaths are available in various sizes with inner diameter ranging from 9.5 to 13 Fr, outer diameter ranging from 12 to 15 Fr and length ranging from 13 cm (pediatric) to 55 cm.

Types

1. Based on construction—Reinforced and nonreinforced
2. Based on length—female/male.

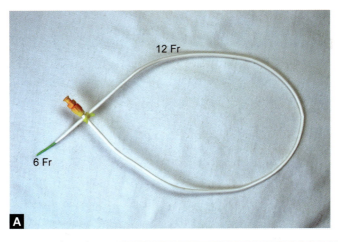

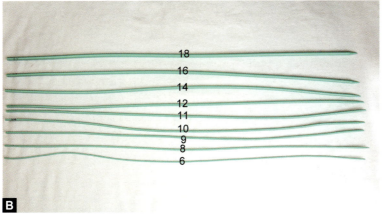

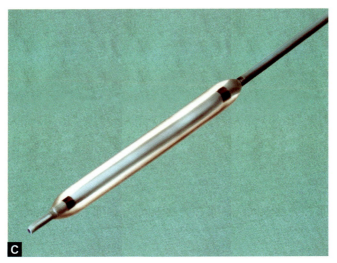

Figures 12A to C: The figure shows the accessories used during ureteroscopy: (A) Nottingham uretheral dilator; (B) Serial teflon ureteral dilator; (C) Balloon ureteral dilator

TABLE 3 Access sheaths specifications

Company	Name	Inner diameter (Fr)	Outer diameter (Fr)	Length (cm)
Cook urological	Cook Flexor	9.5/12/14	11.5/14/16	13/20/28/35/45/55
	Cook Flexor DL	9.5/12	11.5/14	13/20/28/35/45/55
Applied medical resources	Forte	10/12/14	12/14/16	20/28/35/45/55
ACMI corporation	ACMI-Gyrus Uropass®	12	14	24/38/54
Bard	Aquaguide®	12/13	14/15	25/35/45/55

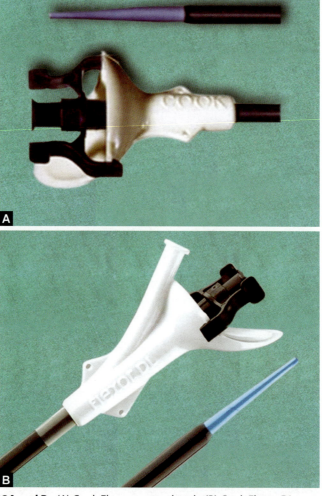

Figures 13A and B: (A) Cook Flexor access sheath; (B) Cook Flexor DL access sheath

Special Types

Dual lumen access sheaths, e.g. Cook flexor DL picture of cross-section, material.

Comparison of Companies

Company	Name	Inner diameter (Fr)	Outer diameter (Fr)	Length (cm)
Cook urological	Cook Flexor	9.5/12/14	11.5/14/16	13/20/28/35/45/55
	Cook Flexor DL	9.5/12	11.5/14	13/20/28/35/45/55
Applied medical resources	Forte	10/12/14	12/14/16	20/28/35/45/55
ACMI corporation	ACMI-Gyrus Uropass®	12	14	24/38/54
Bard	Aquaguide®	12/13	14/15	25/35/45/55

Properties of a Ideal Access Sheath

1. Kink resistant sheath.
2. Hydrophilic coating.
3. Unique hub design.
4. Radiopaque marker band.
5. Dual tapered tip.

PCNL Accessories (Figures 14A and B)

The various accessories used during PCNL help in retrieving stones. The specifications of these accessories are as shown in the Figures 14A and B. The accessories include:

a. Various types of forceps—Broadly the accessories can be classified as:
   - *Triflange*: Requires a larger space to open. Both the biflange and the triflange cannot be easily dismantled.
   - *Biflange*: Requires a smaller space to open.
   - *Aligator*: Requires in a smaller space, hence can be used in compact system.
b. *Suction cannula*: Helps in evacuation of smaller fragments and thus, reducing the operative time.

The top figure shows the two varieties of suction cannulas available.

The bottom figure shows the PCNL graspers in closed and open position. The figures denote the available sizes (6, 9,12 Fr) and the length of the instrument (360 mm).

Alken needle with sheath (Figure 15): 8 Fr needle which is passed over the wire. It does not have sharp cutting edges at the tip. The Alken sheath is 10 Fr, this snuggly fits over the needle. Alken needle length is 26 cm, sheath length is 15 cm. While introduction of the needle the sheath is preintroduced and the needle is passed over the wire. Once the needle reaches the pelvicalyceal system the sheath is advanced into PCS and the needle withdrawn. Sheath is useful to pass a safety guidewire. The guide rod goes through the sheath after which it is withdrawn and the dilatation be start

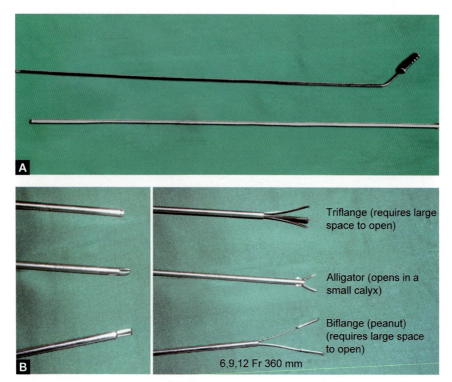

Figures 14A and B: (A) Suction cannula; (B) Various types of forceps used in PCNL

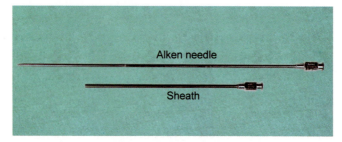

Figure 15: Alken needle

The Alkens needle is also useful to negotiate oblique (zig-zag) tracts or to negotiate through a tough fibrous tissue as it is made up of stainless steel. Alken sheath can also be used to insert antegrade double J stent.

REFERENCES

1. Cook Urology 2010.
2. Cook Urology 2010 Domestic product catalogue pg 23.

3. Cook Urology 2010 Domestic product catalogue pg 15.
4. Cook Urology 2010 Domestic product catalogue pg 18.
5. Cook Urology 2010 Domestic product catalogue pg 22.
6. Cook Urology 2010 Domestic product catalogue pg 25.
7. Cook Urology 2010 Domestic product catalogue pg 20.
8. Cook Urology 2010 Domestic product catalogue pg 14.
9. http://www.terumois.com/products/guidewires/Advantage.aspx accessed on 28/08/2013.
10. Cook Urology 2010 Domestic product catalogue pg 10.
11. http://www.bostonscientific.com/templatedata/imports/Microsite/Stone/collateral/Products_for_Ureteroscopy.pdf accessed on 28/08/2013.
12. Cook Urology 2010 Domestic product catalogue pg 6.
13. Cook Urology 2010 Domestic product catalogue pg 84.
14. Cook Urology 2010 Domestic product catalogue pg 88 (Cook Urology 2010 Domestic product catalogue pg 89).
15. http://www.bostonscientific.com/templatedata/imports/Microsite/Stone/collateral/Percuflex-Brochure.pdf accessed on 28/08/2013.
16. Cook Urology 2010 Domestic product catalogue pg 94.
17. http://www.endotherapeutics.com.au/memokath accessed on 28/08/2013.
18. Indian Journal of Surgery, Vol. 65, No. 5, Sept-Oct, 2003, pp. 405-412 I.Singh.
19. http://www.bostonscientific.com/templatedata/imports/Microsite/Stone/collateral/Retromax-Brochure.pdf accessed on 28/08/2013).
20. Ho CH, Chen SC, Chung SD, Lee YJ, Chen J, Yu HJ, et al. Determining the Appropriate Length of a Double-Pigtail Ureteral Stent by Both Stent Configurations and Related Symptoms. J Endourol. 2008;22:1427-31.
21. Palmer JS, Palmer LS. A simple and reliable formula for determining the proper JJ stent length in the pediatric patient: Age + 10. Urol 2007;70:264.
22. http://www.freedomed.com/types-of-catheters accessed on 22/07/2013.
23. http://www.mountainside-medical.com/products/Red-Rubber-Catheters.html accessed on 22/07/2013.
24. http://www.sportaid.com/bard-red-rubber-catheters-8-22-fr.html. accessed on 22/07/2013.
25. Tatem AE, Klaaseen A, Lewis RW, Terris MK Frederick Eugene Basil Foley: Fredric E.B Foley (1891–1966) His life and innovations Urol 2013;81(5):927-9.
26. http://www.genmedhealth.com/static/Foley_catheter.
27. Cook Urology 2010 Domestic product catalogue pg 60 accessed on 22/07/2013.
28. Cook Urology 2010 Domestic product catalogue pg 58.
29. Cook Urology 2010 Domestic product catalogue pg 61.
30. (http://www.lifebeatonline.com/template data/imports/collateral/Urology/broc_graspit_01_ur_us.pdf accessed on 28/08/2013).
31. Cook Urology 2010 Domestic product catalogue pg 62.
32. (http://www.bostonscientific.com/templatedata/imports/collateral/Urology/spec_gemini_04_us.pdf accessed on 28/08/2013).
33. http://www.lifebeatonline.com/templatedata/imports/collateral/Urology/broc_segura_01_ur_us.pdf accessed on 28/08/2013.
34. Cook Urology 2010 Domestic product catalogue pg 60.

35. (http://www.bostonscientific.com/templatedata/imports/collateral/Urology/broc_stonecone_01_ur_us.pdf accessed on 28/08/2013).
36. http://www.percsys.com/pdfs/Accordion%20CoAx%20Stone%20Control%20Device%2090-0949-01%20rC%201-11.pdf accessed on 28/08/2013.
37. http://www.bostonscientific.com/templatedata/imports/Microsite/Stone/collateral/Backstop-Brochure.pdf accessed on 28/08/2013.

CHAPTER
12

Sterilization

DEFINITIONS

Disinfection and sterilization are necessary to ensure that medical and surgical instruments do not transmit infectious pathogens to patients. The method of sterilization varies from patient-to-patient.

Sterilization is defined as the process by which an article, surface or medium is freed of all living microorganisms either in the vegetative or spore state.

Disinfection means the process that eliminates all pathogenic microorganisms (or in other words organisms capable of giving rise to infection), except bacterial spores, on inanimate objects. A few disinfectants will kill spores with prolonged exposure times (3–12 hours); these are called chemical sterilants.[1]

High-level disinfectants work at similar concentrations but with shorter exposure periods (e.g. 20 minutes for 2% glutaraldehyde), by killing all microrganisms except large numbers of bacterial spore.[1] Intermediate-level disinfectants might destroy mycobacteria, vegetative bacteria, most viruses, and most fungi but do not necessarily kill bacterial spores.[1] Low-level disinfectants can kill most vegetative bacteria, some fungi, and some viruses in a shorter period of time (<10 minutes).[1]

Germicide is an agent that can kill microorganisms, particularly pathogenic organisms ('germs'). Germicides differ markedly, primarily in their antimicrobial spectrum and rapidity of action.[1]

Antiseptics are substances that prevent or arrest the growth or action of microorganisms by inhibiting their activity or by destroying them. Antiseptics are applied to living tissue and skin; disinfectants are antimicrobials applied only to inanimate objects. In general, antiseptics are used only on the skin and not for surface disinfection, and disinfectants are not used for skin antisepsis because they can injure skin and other tissues.[1]

Cleaning is the removal of visible soil (e.g. organic and inorganic material) from objects and surfaces and is usually performed manually or mechanically using water with detergents or enzymatic products.[1]

Decontamination refers to the process of removing pathogenic microorganisms from objects so they are safe to handle, use, or discard.[1]

Approach to Disinfection and Sterilization

Spaulding believed the nature of disinfection could be understood readily if instruments and items for patient care were categorized as critical, semicritical.

He devised a classification system more than 40 years ago which is still in use in most of the international guidelines on sterilization and disinfection including the CDC guideline.[2]

Spauldings Classification[2]

The items were classified as follows:
1. *Critical items*: These were defined as those items which enter the body cavity, vascular system or nonintact mucous membranes. All the surgical instruments are classified as critical. The goal should be to make objects sterile. The preferred method of sterilization is steam sterilization or low temperature sterilization.
2. *Semi critical items*: These are the items which directly or indirectly come in contact with intact mucous membrane or nonintact skin. The aim is to offer high level disinfection which will make the object free of microorganisms except bacterial spores. However, it is always preferable to sterilize semi-critical items whenever they are compatible with available sterilization.
3. *Noncritical items*: These are the items which come in contact with skin but not mucous membrane such as BP cuffs or crutches. The aim is low level disinfection by cleaning.

Different Methods of Sterilization[1,5]

1. Steam sterilization

Mechanism of action: Moist heat causes irreversible coagulation and denaturation of enzymes and structural protein.

Advantages: Nontoxic, easy to control and monitoring, rapidly microbicidal, least affected by organic/inorganic soils, rapid cycle time.

Disadvantages: Heat sensitive instruments cannot be sterilized and repeated sterilization with this technique will lead to loss of sharpness of cutting instruments.

Uses: Critical and semicritical items that are heat and moisture resistant.

Facts and Myths Regarding Steam Sterilization

All instruments (assembled endoscopes) should be opened or unlocked to allow the steam to reach all parts of the instrument. Temperature should be 121°C, with pressure of 106 kPa(15 lb/in 2) for 30 minutes. 20–30 minutes should elapse to permit the sterilizer to cool sufficiently. This ensures complete sterilization.

Myths and Common Procedural Mistakes

1. Not allowing sufficient time hurrying up to get instruments/linen fast thus not achieving enough pressure or exposure time for sterilization.
2. Tight packing of linen in drums does not allow enough steam to circulate.
3. Autoclaved items stored for long time without lid lead to ineffective sterilization.

Following devices may be steam sterilized—rigid telescopes (autoclavable), working elements, trocars/sheaths, reusable thick tubing, 3 L saline bottles, insulated and noninsulated surgical instruments (forceps, scissors, suction tubes, etc.) Sharp instruments are not autoclaved as their sharpness is lost. Wherever possible this method should be used, as it is the cheapest and most reliable method of sterilization.

Dry heat Sterilization is another way to sterilize needles and endoscope instruments. A convection oven with an insulated stainless steel chamber and perforated shelving to allow the circulation of hot air is recommended, but dry heat sterilization can be achieved with a simple oven as long as a thermometer is used to verify the temperature inside the oven. It has got advantages of being an effective procedure even for instruments that cannot be disassembled, protective for sharp instruments, leaving no chemical residue and eliminating wet pack problems in humid climates. The main disadvantage as compared to steam sterilization is requirement of more time, continuous source of electricity besides being contraindicated for plastic and rubber items. Generally, after the desired temperature is reached, timing begins. The following temperature/time ratios are recommended; 170°C 60 minutes 160°C 120 minutes 150°C 150 minutes 140°C 180 minutes depending upon the temperature selected, the total cycle time (preheating, sterilization time and cool down) will range from about 2.5 hours at 170°C to more than 6 hours at 140°C.

Hydrogen Peroxide Gas Plasma Sterilization

Mechanism of action: Destroys by combined use of hydrogen peroxide gas and generation of free radicals (hydroxyl and hydroproxyl free radicals).

Advantages: Nontoxic, cycle time from 35–60 min, simple to operate, most of the instruments can be sterilized.

Disadvantages: Linens cannot be processed, a hydrogen peroxide level more than 1ppm. TWA cannot be processed, it requires special unit for packaging. Plastics and corrosion sensitive metal cannot be processed, expensive, non-compatible with cellulose, smaller units are unable to take large volumes.

Uses: Compatible with most (>95%) medical devices and materials. (laparoscopes, nephroscopes, semirigid and flexible ureteroscopes, cables, etc.).

Myths/Facts and Common Procedural Mistakes in Plasma Sterilization

Plasma sterilization: This method uses 1.8 milliliters of 58% hydrogen peroxide, which is vaporized, in a sterilization chamber. The vapor is converted into plasma through the use of radio frequency (RF) energy. Plasma consists of highly charged particles and free radicals to sterilize instruments in about one hour without producing toxic residues or emissions. Commercially, marketed as STERRAD™ (Figure 1).

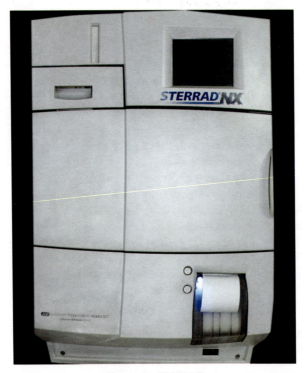

Figure 1: STERRAD

It is useful to sterilize almost everything such as rigid telescopes, flexible fiberscopes and semi-rigid fiberscopes, video cameras, fiber- and fluid-light cables, surgical instruments, insulated (forceps, scissors, etc.), surgical instruments, noninsulated (forceps, scissors, etc.), high frequency, cords etc.

Ethylene Oxide sterilization (ETO)

Mechanism of action: Alkylation of protein, DNA, and RNA
Advantages: Penetrates packaging materials, device lumens, user friendly and compatible with most medical devices.

Disadvantages: Requires time for preparation, ETO is toxic, a carcinogen, and flammable, Lengthy cycle/aeration time.

Uses: Critical items (and sometimes semicritical items) that are moisture or heat sensitive and cannot be sterilized by steam sterilization.

Facts/Myths for ETO Sterilization

Ethylene oxide (EO or ETO) gas is commonly used to sterilize objects sensitive to temperatures greater than 60°C such as plastics, laparoscopes, endoscopic lens, wires, and electric items, etc. Ethylene oxide treatment is generally carried out between 30°C and 60°C with relative humidity above 30% and a gas concentration between 200 and 800 mg/L for at least three hours. Ethylene oxide penetrates well, moving through paper, cloth, and some plastic films and is highly effective. ETO can kill all known viruses, bacteria and fungi, including bacterial spores and is satisfactory for most medical materials, even with repeated use. However, it is highly flammable, and requires a longer time to sterilize than any heat treatment. The process also requires a period of post-sterilization aeration to remove toxic residues. Ethylene oxide is the most common sterilization method, used for over 70% of total sterilizations, and for 50% of all disposable medical devices.

Instruments frequently gas sterilized in urology practice include: Fiberoptic endoscopes, surgical telescopes, laparoscope, plastic instruments (e.g. specula, syringes), anesthesia masks and circuits, rubber and plastic tubing (e.g. catheters), respirators and inhalation therapy supplies.

Problem: It is the best and relatively cheapest method of sterilization. But takes long time. Poststerilization aeration does not make it useful on day-to-day basis.

Chemical Agents Used as Disinfectants/Sterilants

Chemical solutions are accepted 'liquid chemical sterilizing agents', provided that the immersion time is sufficiently long.

*Alcohol (*ethyl alcohol, isopropyl alcohol, (60–90% solutions in water)

Mechanism of action: Denaturation of proteins.

Advantages: Easily available, no activation time.

Disadvantages: Lacks sporicidal action, damage the shellac mountings of lensed instruments, tends to swell and harden rubber and plastic, flammable.

Uses: To disinfect external surfaces of equipment (e.g. stethoscopes, ventilators, manual ventilation bags), and ultrasound instruments.

Aldehyde group of chemical disinfectants (glutaraldehyde (2.4%) and formaldehyde).

Mechanism of action: Alkylation of sulfhydryl enzymes and Amino acid (AA)

Advantage: Relatively inexpensive and compatible with most of the instruments.

Disadvantages: Respiratory irritation from glutaraldehyde vapor, Pungent and irritating odor. Relatively slow mycobactericidal activity. Coagulates blood and fixes tissue to surfaces. Allergic contact dermatitis.

Uses: Formaldehyde preparation of viral vaccines, to preserve specimens, to disinfect fluid pathways in dialysis machines.

Glutaraldehyde

High level disinfectant for Endoscopes, laparoscopic trocars.
Myths and problems with gluteraldehyde and formaldehyde as disinfectants.

Glutaraldehyde (Cidex) Sterilization

Decontaminate, clean, and thoroughly dry all instruments and other items to be sterilized. Water from wet items will dilute the chemical solution, thereby reducing its effectiveness. Prepare the glutaraldehyde-containing solution (or other chemical solution) by following the manufacturer's instructions. After preparing the solution, put it in a clean container with a lid (Figure 2). Always mark the container with the date the solution was prepared and the date it expires. (Usually 2 weeks). Open all hinged instruments and other items and disassemble those with sliding or multiple parts. The solution must contact all surfaces in order for sterilization to be achieved. Completely submerge all instruments and other items in the solution. All parts of the items should be under the surface of the solution. For sterilization, 10–12 hrs of soakage is required. After that, instruments should be cleaned by sterile water, as glutaraldehyde is toxic to the endothelium.

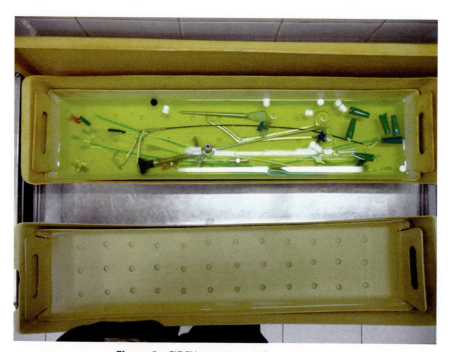

Figure 2: CIDEX container with instruments

Product Description

- 2.45% w/v glutaraldehyde with activator.
- It is available in a 1, 2 and 5 liter package. The use life is 14 days.

MYTHS

Cidex is commonly used for rapid sterilization. Instruments are soaked only for 20–30 minutes. This achieves only disinfection. Telescopes if soaked for 12 hours may cause damage of cement resulting in fogging of telescopes. Even other instrument's life may be reduced with long soakage. Thus it is myth that cidex sterilizes instruments, it only disinfects!!

For it to be effective, instruments should be cleaned thoroughly preferably by enzymatic solution it is hardly ever done thus severely compromising even the disinfection process.

All instruments should be dissembled. Many of our scopes cannot be dissembled; all joints cannot be separated thus further compromising disinfection process.

Instruments are taken in out several times resulting into dilution thereby further reducing efficacy of solution.

Not covering by lid continuously and no monitoring of pH. Thus not knowing about effectiveness of solution.

Thus, cidex, the way in which it is commonly used is nothing but eyewash and far from sterilization.

Formaldehyde

One of the curious applications of this agent, prevalent in surgical operation theaters in India, is in the form of tablets for the sterilization of delicate instruments that can be damaged by heat. These are available in the form of Para formaldehyde polymer of formaldehyde, as tablets of one gram each. A literature search did not provide adequate information regarding the efficacy of this form of formaldehyde in sterilization. This form of sterilization is already discarded from almost all countries. One Indian study suggested that exposure of formaldehyde vapors for at least 24 hours in airtight compartment may result in sterilization. However, this recommendation is on personal experience and not evidence based.

Myths: Formalin tablets are kept in Acrylic box containing scopes. No standardization about no of tablets, duration of exposure, how many times the door of box is opened, when to change the tablets, etc. Thus most common method of instrument sterilization adopted in private practice is the one, which is obsolete...!!

Orthophthalaldehyde (OPA)

Mechanism of action: Interacts with AA, proteins to cause their breakdown.

Advantages: Fast acting high-level disinfectant. No activation required. Nonirritant.

Excellent materials compatibility. Does not coagulate blood or fix tissues to surfaces. High stability over a wide pH range.

Disadvantages: Stains skin, mucous membranes, clothing, and environmental surfaces.

Repeated exposure may result in hypersensitivity in some patients with bladder cancer. More expensive than glutaraldehyde. Eye irritation. Slow sporicidal activity.

Uses: High level disinfectant for endoscopes, anesthesia equipment, laparoscopic trocars.

Pack size-1 liter and 5 liter. The shelf life is 2 years for unopened bottle and 75 days for open bottle (provided they have not extended beyond expiry). Test strips are used to determine minimum effective concentration (MEC). The Cidex OPA strips are used to determine the use life (up to 14 days). OPA does not require activator.[3]

Per Acetic Acid

Mechanism of action: Oxidizing agent which denatures protein, disrupts cell wall and oxidizes sulfhydryl group.

Advantages: Rapid sterilization cycle time (30–45 minutes). Low temperature (50–55°C) sterilization. Environmental friendly by-products (acetic acid, O_2, H_2O). Fully automated.

Disadvantage: Potential material incompatibility (e.g. aluminum anodized coating becomes dull).

Used for immersible instruments only. Only one scope or a small number of instruments can be processed in a cycle. Serious eye and skin damage (concentrated solution) with contact. Point-of-use system, no sterile storage.[4]

Uses

Automated machine used to sterilize medical instruments (Laparoscopes, endoscopes), surgical instruments, dental instruments.

Iodophors

Mechanism: Disruption of protein and nucleic acid structure and synthesis by iodine.

Advantages: Nonstaining, easily available, relatively inexpensive.

Disadvantages: High level disinfectant, adversely affect silicone tubing and hence should not be used on silicone catheters, cannot be used as hard surface disinfectants due to concentration differences.

Uses: Used as antiseptics, disinfecting blood culture bottles and medical equipment such as thermometers, endoscopes, etc.

Hydrogen Peroxide

Mechanism: Active hydroxyl free radicals destroy membrane lipids, DNA, etc.
Advantages: No activation required. May enhance removal of organic matter and organisms. No disposal issues. No odor or irritation issues. Does not coagulate blood or fix tissues to surfaces.
Disadvantages: Material compatibility concerns (brass, zinc, copper, and nickel/silver plating) both cosmetic and functional. Serious eye damage with contact.
Uses: Disinfection of ventilators, contact lenses, endoscopes. Occasionally used in catheter bags to eliminate bag as source of bladder bacteriuria and contamination.

STEPS OF STERILIZATION AND PROCESSING OF SURGICAL INSTRUMENTS

Precleaning: Gross soil (blood, sputum) should be removed at point of use. If cleaning not possible then submerge instruments in detergent/enzymatic cleaner to prevent organic matter from drying.
Disassembly: Facilitates the access of cleaning agent to the device surfaces.
Cleaning: Cleaning is the removal of foreign material (e.g. soil, and organic material) from objects and is normally accomplished using water with detergents or enzymatic products. Thorough cleaning is required before high-level disinfection and sterilization because inorganic and organic materials that remain on the surfaces of instruments interfere with the effectiveness of these processes. Cleaning is done either manually or mechanically. With manual cleaning, the two essential components are friction and fluidics. Friction (e.g. rubbing/scrubbing the soiled area with a brush) (Figure 3) and Fluidics (i.e. fluids under pressure) (Figures 4A and B) are used to remove soil and debris from internal channels. The most common types of mechanical or automatic cleaners are ultrasonic cleaners, washer-decontaminators, washer-disinfectors, and washer-sterilizers.

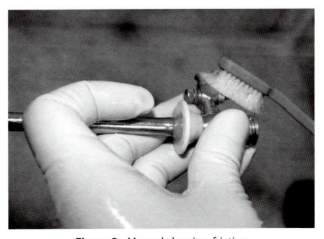

Figure 3: Manual cleaning-friction

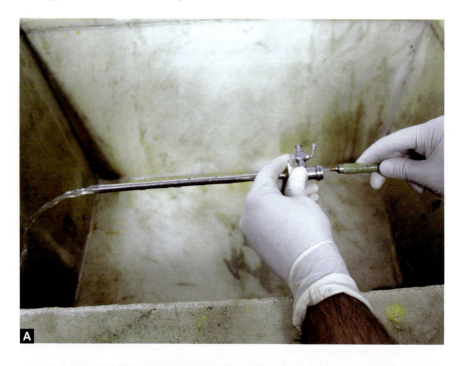

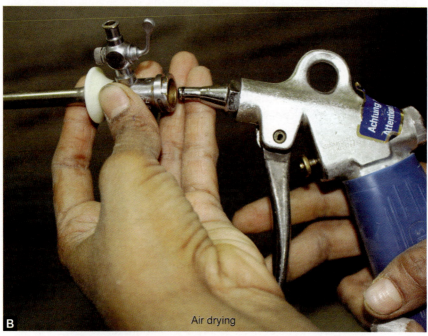

Figures 4A and B: (A) Manual cleaning fluidics; (B) Air drying

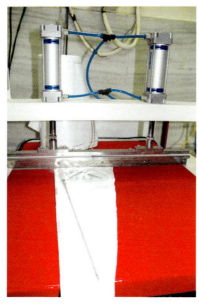

Figure 5: Packaging for sterilization

Packaging: Once cleaned and dried, instruments requiring sterilization must be wrapped or placed in rigid containers and should be arranged in instrument trays/baskets. Options include peel open pouches, roll stock/reels and sterilization wraps.

Loading: In perforated trays for free circulation of sterilizing steam/agent to ensure proper exposure of all instruments.

Sterilization process: According to the type of instruments/devices to be sterilized.

Storage: Shelf life varies according to the porosity of the packaging material and storage conditions. Heat-sealed (Figure 5), plastic peel-down pouches in 3-mil (3/1000 inch) polyethylene overwrap have been reported to be sterile for as long as 9 months after sterilization whereas the double layer muslin covering can keep the contents sterile for a period of 1 month.

Monitoring: It is done by using a combination of mechanical, chemical, and biological indicators to evaluate the sterilizing conditions and indirectly the microbiologic status of the processed items. Biological indicators are considered to be the ideal monitors of the sterilization process because they measure the sterilization process directly by using the most resistant microorganisms (i.e., *Bacillus* spores). Chemical monitors are either heat-or chemical-sensitive inks that change color when one or more sterilization parameters (e.g., steam-time, temperature; ETO-time) are present and they should be preferably placed on the inside of the pack too.

Sterilization of Individual Instruments

The various instructions for sterilization vary with manufacturers. The following are general guidelines for various instruments and assembly:

TURP Instruments—Spaulding-high Level Disinfection or Sterilization

Predisinfection: Separate the cable from the working element immediately after use, remove the telescope immerse the various parts of the assembly in a disinfectant solution.

Cleaning: The working element should be separated from the high frequency cord and rinsed with tap water. The basic principle after cleaning is to ensure that the hollow tubes are dry. This can be accomplished with a brush and dry cotton swab. In this assembly the telescope channel and the electrode channel should be cleaned thoroughly. Special care should be taken to avoid damage of the insulation.

Disinfection: The parts are again placed in a disinfectant solution (glutaraldehyde), following which the instruments are again rinsed and dried.

Sterilization

a. Telescope—autoclavable, plasma, ETO
b. Working element—autoclavable, plasma sterilization
c. High frequency cord, ETO, sterrad (glutaldehyde)
d. Sheath—autoclavable, plasma sterilization
e. Loops, plasma sterilization, ETO
f. Light cable—sterrad, ETO
   The color code knob and the plastic ring tend to get worn off with repeated uses. Either with gas or steam sterilization.

Sterilization of Ureteroscopes-semicritical item- Recommended High Level Disinfection

Decontamination: Allow the instrument to soak in a disinfectant and cleaning solution. This helps to get rid of the microorganisms and detach the residual clots and debris over the instrument. Prior to cleaning the light cable should be detached from the instrument.

Cleaning: This can be done by holding the instrument under running tap water and with the help of a pressure injector or a brush. The parts in the ureteroscope which should be especially taken care of are the eyepiece, objective lens, light cable entry point (see figure). Thereafter the instrument should be meticulously dried.

Sterilization: Steam or gas sterilization.

Sterilization of Accessories

Decontamination: These instruments after sterilization should be kept immediately in a disinfectant or cleaning solution.

Cleaning: This step is critical because any residual debris renders the ensuing steps useless. However, one should ensure that the insulation and other protective coatings do not come off. The accessories can be cleaned with a ultrasound cleaner. Care should be particularly taken to keep all the hinges and joint open, instruments being completely immersed, the channels can be flushed with cleaning gun. Thereafter the channels should be dried inside and out.

Sterilization

a. Baskets—ETO, plasma (cannot be autoclaved)
b. Dilator sets—ETO, plasma
c. Alken dilators—autoclavable, ETO, plasma
d. Percutaneous nephrolithotomy (PCNL) forceps—autoclavable, ETO, plasma
e. Energy probes—autoclavable, ETO, plasma
f. Ultrasonography (USG) probe—autoclaved.

Sterilization of Laparoscopic Instruments

- Insulated instruments-autoclave
- Ports-metal-autoclavable, sterrad or ETO
- Scissors-blunts the sharpness in autoclave
- Retracting instruments-autoclave
- Camera-sterad, some cameras glutaraldehyde
- Nephroscopes-autoclavable (Hopkins 2). All Hopkin 2 telescope are autoclavable
- Ureteroscopes-autoclavable
- Flexible URS-ETO, H_2O_2 (glutaraldehyde).

Salient Features for Sterilization of Cystoscopes and Telescopes

Autoclavable telescopes can be sterilized with autoclaving. If a nonautoclavable telescope (used in the past) is autoclaved, the metals and the glass items would expand unequally, as the temperature would decrease and the external surface cooled the metals would shrink to its normal size. This phenomenon was described on the basis of the principle of coefficient of expansion. In the older version of telescopes the coefficient of expansion would vary and they would expand and shrink at different rates, thus the rod lens would expand but the metal sheath covering would not expand thus leading to breakage. This shortcoming is overcome with the advent of autoclavable telescopes.

Telescopes can be sterilized in glutaraldehyde. The telescopes need to be kept for over 12 hours for the same. Prolonged insertion can at times leads to fogging. The surgeon should specifically look for cracks on the sheath prior to insertion in glutaraldehyde. The other methods of sterilization include hydrogen peroxide and ethylene oxide sterilization.

Tips and Tricks in Sterilizing

Since cystoscope accessories except the telescope are made up of metal, they can be autoclaved. The plastic rings for color coding get damaged during the sterilization. The sheaths can be disinfected (high level) with glutaraldehyde, or can be sterilized by hydrogen peroxide. Before placing the instrument in formalin chamber it is necessary to clean the inner and outer wall with water, following this they should be completely dried, in order to prevent corrosive action of formaldehyde with water. Prolonged insertion of the instrument in water particularly in hard water results in deposition of crystals. The crystals lead to malfunction of the inlet/outlet taps. The taps can be periodically dismantled and cleaned to prevent this. Formaldehyde reacts with water and forms formic acid, which gives black discoloration to the instrument. The summary of sterilization methods are listed in Table 1.

TABLE 1: Summary of sterilization methods

	Autoclave	Plasma sterilization	ETO
TURP instruments	See text	See text	See text
Telescope	Yes	Yes	Yes
Working element	Yes	Yes	Yes
Loops	No	Yes	Yes
High frequency cord	No	Yes	Yes
Light cable	No	Yes	Yes
PCNL instruments	See text	See text	See text
Amplatz dilator	No	Yes	Yes
Metallic dilator	Yes	Yes	Yes
Percutaneous nephrolithotomy (PCNL) forceps	Yes	Yes	Yes
Energy probe	No	Yes	Yes
Laparoscopic instruments			
Metal ports	Yes	Yes	Yes
Scissors	No	Yes	Yes

REFERENCES

1. Guideline for Disinfection and Sterilization in Healthcare Facilities, 2008, CDC (Centers for Disease Control and prevention).
2. Spaulding EH. Chemical disinfection of medical and surgical materials. In: Lawrence C, Block SS (Eds). Disinfection, sterilization, and preservation. Philadelphia: Lea and Febiger; 1968.pp.517-31.
3. Russell AD. Bacterial resistance to disinfectants: present knowledge and future problems. J Hosp Infect 1998;43:S57-68.
4. Rutala WA, Weber DJ. Clinical effectiveness of low-temperature sterilization technologies. Infect Control Hosp Epidemiol 1998;19:798-804.
5. Rutala WA, Weber DJ. Disinfection of endoscopes: review of new chemical sterilants used for high-level disinfection. Infect Control Hosp Epidemiol 1999;20:69-76.

CHAPTER

13

Open Urology Instruments

OPEN SURGERY RETRACTORS

Bookwalter Retractor (Figure 1)

Bookwalter retractor includes:
- Table post
- Horizontal bar
- 1" post coupling
- Medium oval ring
- 2" × 6" malleable retractors (2 ea.)
  51 mm × 152 mm
- 2" × 3" kelly retractors (2 ea.)
  51 mm × 76 mm
- 2" × 4" Kelly retractor
  51 mm × 101 mm
- Balfour retractor
- Ratchet mechanisms (2 ea.)
- Tilt Ratchet mechanisms (6 ea.)
- Segmented ring
- 11/2" × 6" Malleable retractor
  38 mm × 152 mm
- 3" × 6" Malleable retractor
  76 mm × 152 mm
- 2" × 5" Kelly retractor
  51 mm × 127 mm
- 2" × 6" Kelly retractor
  51 mm × 152 mm
- Horizontal flex bar
- Harrington retractor
- Gelpi retractor

As the retractors are fixed to the bar on OT table, the assistant need not hold the retractor.

Retractors are available in various shape and sizes for special surgeries, e.g. and renal cell carcinoma (RCC) with inferior vena cava (IVC) thrombus, large renal tumor, retroperitoneal lymph node (RPLND).

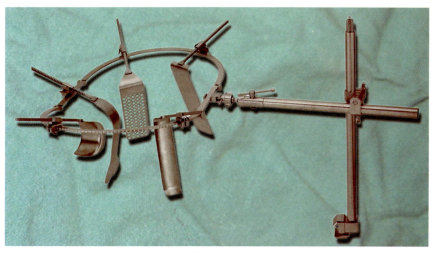

Figure 1: Bookwalter retractor

Disadvantage: Bars might be a cause of obstacle for assistant to stand and see the surgery.

Denis Brown Abdominal Retractor (Figure 2)

Denis Brown abdominal retractor with:
- 2 blade 40 × 30 mm
- 2 blade 40 × 40 mm include
- 1 frame 190 × 160 mm
- Used in any abdominal surgery for retraction and pediatric surgery.

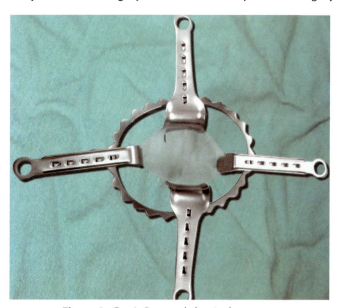

Figure 2: Denis Brown abdominal retractor

Millin's Self-retaining Bladder Retractor with a Provision for Attachment of Third Blade (Figure 3)

Two blades are fitted on horizontal bars which can slide and may be fixed by screws. In between these two blades there is another screw which may attach the third blade when required. When finger bows are separated the blades are lying closer. When finger bows are approximated the blades are separated.

This retractor is used during transvesical prostatectomy. The third blade retracts the fundus of the bladder. This keeps the bladder wide open and allows proper inspection of the prostate cavity and hemostasis under vision.

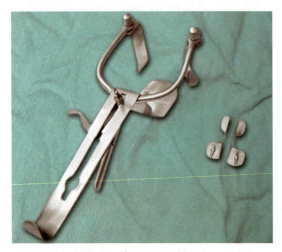

Figure 3: Millin's self-retaining bladder retractor

Ring Retractor (Figures 4A and B)

- Turner Warwick retractor set, consisting of ONE circular ring 23 cm, four blades angled with lip 114 mm × 60 mm and four blades curved 51 mm × 38 mm
- Used during urethroplasty for adequate exposure of the perineum.

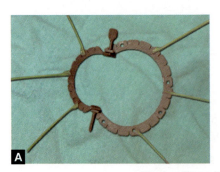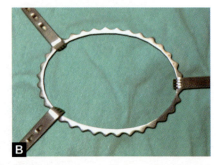

Figures 4A and B: Ring retractor

Gilvernet Hilar Retractor (Figure 5A)

- Used for retraction of vein, renal hilum.
- Available in various sizes; 20 cm (8 mm, 15 mm, 20 mm and 23 mm)
- After creating plane of gilvernet it can be used for retraction of tissues at renal hilum.

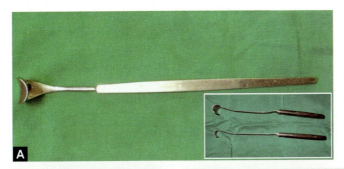

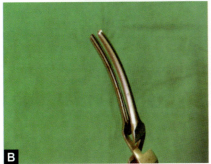
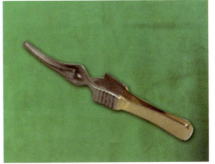

Figures 5A and B: A. Gilvernet hilar retractor; B. Bulldog clamp

VASCULAR INSTRUMENTS

A. *Bulldog clamp (Figure 5B)*: It is used to grip blood vessels. DeBakey Bulldog clamps, cross-action, 1 × 2 vascular teeth. Shape: Straight and curved material used: Stainless steel.
Various sizes: 1.5", 2", 2.5", 3"

Straight

- *Jaw length*: 20 mm, 30 mm, 45 mm, 65 mm.
- *Total length*: 79 mm, 89 mm, 105 mm, 127 mm.

Curved

- *Jaw length*: 20 mm, 30 mm, 45 mm, 65 mm
- *Total length*: 76 mm, 86 mm, 105 mm, 121 mm
- B. *Satinsky vascular clamp (Figure 6)*:
- Satinsky classic vena cava clamps.

- 1 × 2 vascular teeth satinsky vascular clamp used to primarily clamp blood vessels.
- *Material used*: Stainless steel.
- Dimensions (inch) L x W x H: 11.1 × 3.8 × 2.0
- *Various sizes*: 8", 9", 10"

Jaw length	68 mm	63 mm	57 mm
Jaw depth	12 mm	9 mm	6 mm
Total length	241 mm	241 mm	241 mm

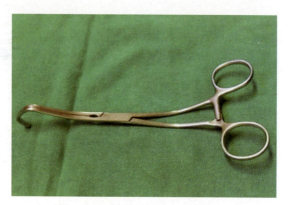

Figure 6: Satinsky vascular clamp

B. *Cooley vascular clamp (Figure 7)*:
- Cooley *classic anastomosis clamps*
- Blades calibrated at 5 mm intervals, 2 × 2 vascular teeth.
- *Dimensions (inch) L × W × H*: 7.0 × 3.0 × 0.25
- *Jaw length*: 73 mm
- *Jaw depth*: 17 mm
- *Total length*: 254 mm

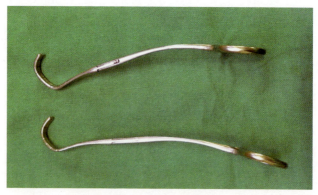

Figure 7: Cooley vascular clamp

D. *DeBakey vascular clamps (Figure 8)*:
- DeBakey Classic Multi-Purpose Clamps,
- 60° angle, 1 × 2 vascular teeth.
- *Dimensions (inch) L × W × H*: 7.0 × 3.0 × 0.25
- *Jaw length*: 40 mm, 50 mm, 70 mm, 100 mm
- *Total length*: 244 mm, 203 mm, 241 mm, 305 mm

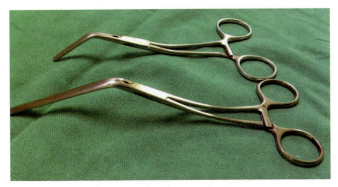

Figure 8: DeBakey vascular clamps

E. *DeBakey vascular forceps (Figure 9)*: DeBakey forcep is used to hold vascular vessels and tissues.

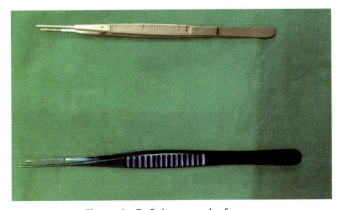

Figure 9: DeBakey vascular forceps

F. *Lambert-Kay vascular IVC clamp (Figure 10)*:
- 1 × 2 vascular teeth
- *Jaw length*: 51 mm
- *Jaw depth*: 20 mm
- *Total length*: 191 mm

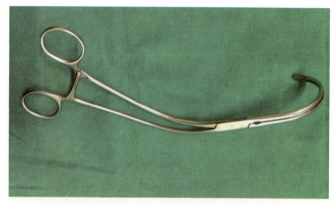

Figure 10: Lambert-Kay vascular IVC clamp

USES OF VASCULAR INSTRUMENTS

- Used for temporary clamping of large vascular structures: iliac vessels, IVC, Aorta, renal artery.
- Also used (bulldog clamp) during creation of A-V fistula.

STONE HOLDING FORCEPS

A. *Desjardins forceps (Figures 11A and B)*: This is a long and slender instrument. There are finger bows but no catch. The shafts are curved, in some it is gentle curve and in other varieties there are different degrees of curvature. The blades are flat and fenestrated centrally. There are no fenestrations in the blade.

It is used during removal of kidney, ureteric or bladder stones.

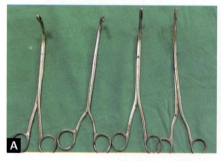 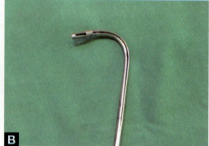

Figures 11A and B: Desjardins forceps

B. *Thompson Walker suprapubic cystolithotomy forceps (Figure 12)*: This forceps consists of finger bows—one finger bow for the thumb is ring like, the other finger bow meant for other fingers is hook like, a pair of shaft and a pair of blades. The blades are longer and the inner surfaces of the blades are provided with fine knobs which help in better gripping of stones. There are no ratchets in this instrument.

USE

Used for suprapubic cystolithotomy. After the bladder is opened by a suprapubic cystotomy the instrument is inserted into the bladder and the stone is removed.

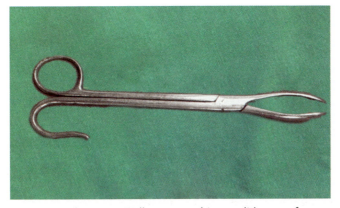

Figure 12: Thompson Walker suprapubic cystolithotomy forceps

INSTRUMENTS USED IN URETHRAL SURGERY

Chisel and Gouge (Figure 13B)

Used in progressive perineal urethroplasty during the step of inferior pubectomy.
- **Gouges (Figure 13A)**
  - Length 8″ (203 mm)
  - 1 ¼″ (32 mm)
- **Hammer**
  - Diameter 1 ½″ (38 mm)
  - Length 7″ (178 mm)
  - Weight 15 oz. (420 g)

Uses: Inferior pubectomy/exicision of callous in transpubic urethroplasty.

Gauge has a curved U-shaped tip which helps in removing the chip of the bone, during pubectomy.

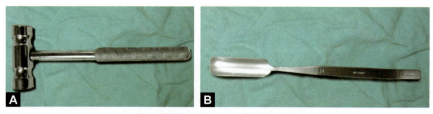

Figures 13A and B: Hammer and gouge

Dilators

- **Metallic bougie:** Characteristics

Clutton's metallic bougie (Figures 14A and B): This is a solid cylindrical metallic instrument. The handle is violin shaped with a long shaft and the terminal end has a smooth curve with a blunt tip. The denominator number denotes the circumference in mm. at the base and the numerator denotes the circumference in mm at tip. This is available in a set of twelve and the different numbers are 6/10, 8/12, 10/14, 12/16….28/32.

Lister's metallic bougie (Figures 14A and B): This is identical to a Clutton's metallic bougie. The differences are—The handle is rounded and the tip is olive pointed. The number written has a difference of three and has the same implication as in Clutton's metallic bougie. This is also available in a set.

Uses of Metallic Bougie

- Used for dilatation of urethra in urethral stricture.
- Used for dilatation of urethra prior to introduction of cystoscope.
- Used during repair of rupture urethra by rail road technique.
- Used for progressive perineal urethroplasty for identification of urethra.

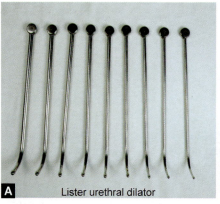

Lister urethral dilator

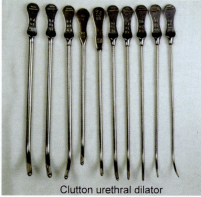

Clutton urethral dilator

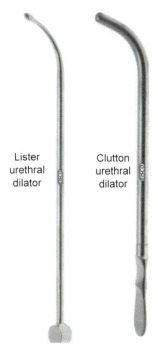

Lister
urethral
dilator

Clutton
urethral
dilator

B

Figures 14A and B: Lister's and Clutton's dilators. Lister's olive end with coin-shaped upper end with size marked. The upper figure is for tip and lower the broad part, Clutton's round ended with violin-shaped upper end 3/6 size marked in millimeters upper for tip 4/8 for broad part. Both are used for dilating male urethra

Haygrove Sound (Figures 15A and B)

Haygrove sound is introduced into the suprapubic sinus and through the bladder neck to the distal limits of the posterior urethra.

Disadvantage: May go into false passage.

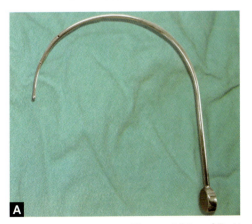

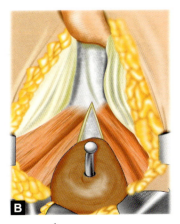

A

B

Figures 15A and B: Haygrove sound

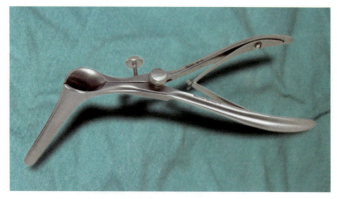

Figure 16: Kilian septum speculum

- **Kilian septum speculum (Figure 16)**
  Total length: 5 1/4" (133 mm)
With variable:
- *Blade length*: 2" (51 mm)
- *Blade length*: 2 1/2" (63 mm)
- *Blade length*: 3" (76 mm)
  Used during perineal urethrostomy, ventral onlay for buccal mucosal graft suturing at proximal urethra.
- **Thudicum (Figure 17)**
  – The speculum is available in a wide range of other sizes, from size 0 to size 7.
  – Size 70 mm
  – Used during perineal uretherostomy
  – Used for proper exposure of proximal urethra.

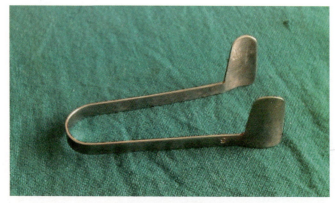

Figure 17: Thudicum

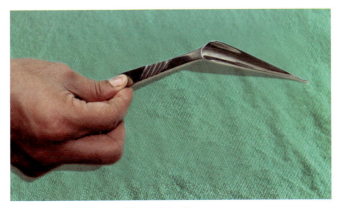

Figure 18: Gorget

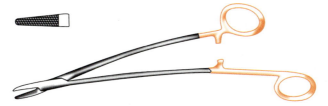

Figure 19: Turner warwick

- **Gorget:** Used for taking sutures from proximal urethra (Figure 18).
- **Turner warwick needle holder:** It is a articulated needle holder. Thumb grip is at an angle to finger grip. Tip of the needle holder holding the needle is always visible. While taking suture from posterior urethra surgeon can always see direction of the needle (Figure 19).

DEFLUX

Deflux is a sterile, highly viscous gel of dextranomer microspheres (50 mg/mL) in a carrier gel of nonanimal stabilized hyaluronic acid (15 mg/mL), constituting a biocompatible and biodegradable implant. The dextranomer microspheres range in size between 80–250 microns with an average size of about 130 microns.

Deflux is supplied prefilled in a 1 mL syringe with a luer lock fitting, and is intended for single use only. The syringe is equipped with a tip cap, plunger and plunger rod. The syringe is terminally sterilized.

Indications

Deflux is indicated for treatment of children with vesicoureteral reflux (VUR) grades II–IV.

Contraindications

Deflux is contraindicated in patients with any of the following conditions:
- Nonfunctional kidney(s)
- Hutch diverticulum
- Ureterocele
- Active voiding dysfunction
- Ongoing urinary tract infection.

It is recommended to use the Deflux metal needle (3.7F x 23G tip x 350 mm) for safe and accurate administration of Deflux. The needle is introduced through 4 French working channel.

The needle is introduced under the bladder mucosa 2–3 mm below the refluxing ureteral orifice at a 6 o'clock position. The needle tip is positioned just under the urothelium and is advanced 4–5 mm in the submucosal plane of the ureter. Deflux is then injected until a prominent bulge appears, and the orifice has assumed a crescent-like shape. Only a small volume (0.5–1.0 mL) is needed to create a sufficient bolus (Figure 1).

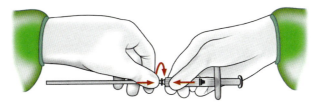

Figure 1: Attachment of Deflux injection needle

PEDIATRIC ENDOUROLOGY INSTRUMENTS

Pediatric Operating Cystoscope—Urethroscope

8/9.5 Fr with Angled Eyepiece (Figures 2A and B)

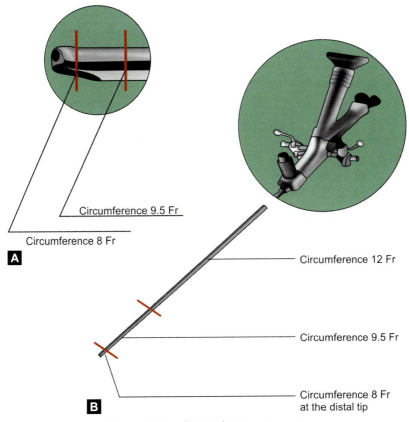

Circumference 9.5 Fr

Circumference 8 Fr

A

Circumference 12 Fr

Circumference 9.5 Fr

Circumference 8 Fr
at the distal tip

B

Figures 2A and B: Pediatric cystoscope

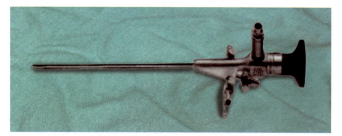

Figure 3: 9.5 Fr scope with forward oblique telescope 30°

8 Fr, 6°, 1 step, 8–12 Fr, length 13 cm, autoclavable, with angled eyepiece, fiber optic light transmission incorporated with, 2 lateral irrigation ports and 1 working channel, 5 Fr. For operating instruments 4 Fr.

9.5 Fr Scope with forward-oblique Telescope 30° (Figure 3)

9.5 Fr, fiber optic light transmission incorporated, 3 Fr working channel and autoclavable.

Instruments for use with Pediatric Operating Cystoscope-Urethroscope 9.5 Fr

- Hook electrode-unipolar, 3 Fr (Figure 4)
- Grasping forceps (Figure 5)

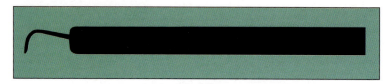

Figure 4: Hook electrode-unipolar, 3 Fr

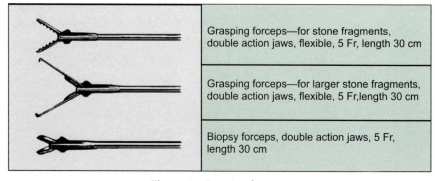

	Grasping forceps—for stone fragments, double action jaws, flexible, 5 Fr, length 30 cm
	Grasping forceps—for larger stone fragments, double action jaws, flexible, 5 Fr, length 30 cm
	Biopsy forceps, double action jaws, 5 Fr, length 30 cm

Figure 5: Grasping forceps

Pediatric Cystoscope-urethro-fiberscope (Figures 6 to 8)

With positive (or logical) deflection, a downward movement of the lever mechanism causes an upward movement of the endoscope tip, and vice versa. Reverse this orientation by choosing the contrapositive mechanism; a downward movement of lever mechanism now causes a downward movement of the endoscope tip.

Positive Deflection Mechanism

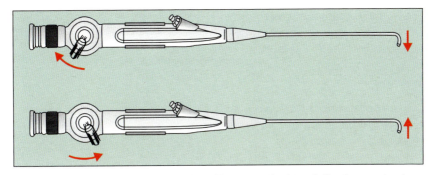

Figure 6: Pediatric cystoscope-urethro-fiberscope: Positive deflection mechanism

Contrapositive Deflection Mechanism

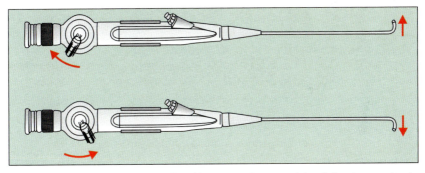

Figure 7: Pediatric cystoscope-urethro-fiberscope: Contrapositive deflection mechanism

A larger angle upward from 270° and downward from 270° allows for the intuitive orientation and visualization of the entire renal tract, including the intrarenal collecting system.

The new angulation mechanism makes it possible to use 200 µ laser fibers without compromising the angulation properties. Even large 365 µ laser fibers only result in a 10% loss of the angulation properties.

Diagnostic and Therapeutic Indications for the Ureteral and Renal Tract

- Lithotripsy and stone extraction in ureteral and renal tract
- Maximum angle of 270° permits access to the entire renal tract, including lower renal calyces
- Allows detection of pathology in anatomical areas difficult to access.

Diagnosis

- Identifying causes of hematuria
- Differential diagnosis of filling defects
- Diagnosis of ureteral tumors.

Therapy

- Removing calculi or foreign bodies
- Treating ureteral tumors
- Coagulating hemorrhagic
- Disintegrating ureteral calculi.

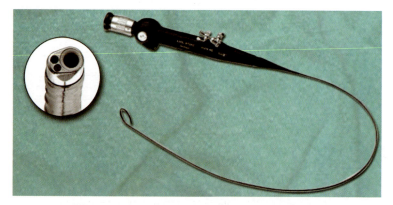

Figure 8: Pediatric cystoscope-urethro-fiberscope

Deflection of distal tip		Direction of view	Angle of view	Working length	Working channel inner diameter	Sheath size
Positive deflection		0°	88°	45 cm	3.6 Fr	7.5 Fr
With Contrapositive deflection		0°	88°	45 cm	3.6 Fr	7.5 Fr

Accessories used with pediatric cystoscope-urethro-fiberscope (Figure 9)

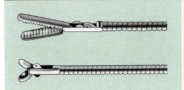

1. Grasping forceps—double action jaws, flexible, 3 Fr, length 60 cm
2. Biopsy forceps—double action jaws, flexible, 3 Fr, length 60 cm

Figure 9: Accessories used with pediatric cystoscope-urethro-fiberscope

Neonatal Cystoscope-Urethroscope 7/9 Fr (Figure 10)

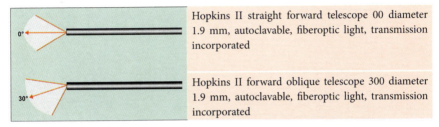

Hopkins II straight forward telescope 00 diameter 1.9 mm, autoclavable, fiberoptic light, transmission incorporated

Hopkins II forward oblique telescope 300 diameter 1.9 mm, autoclavable, fiberoptic light, transmission incorporated

Figure 10: Neonate cystoscope-urethroscope 7/9 Fr

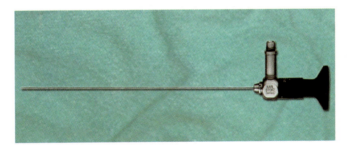

Figure 11: Miniature straight forward telescope 0°, diameter 1.2 mm, length 20 cm, autoclavable, fiber optic light transmission incorporated

Pediatric Operating Cystoscope-urethroscope with Straight Forward Telescope 0° (Figure 11)

- 8/9 Fr.

Special features

- Distal end of sheath is shaping on atraumation runner atraumatically shaped
- Two lateral, right angled irrigation ports
- Minimal sheath diameter
- The wide working channel allows use of 4–5 Fr rigid instruments
- Autoclavable.

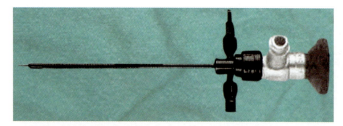

Figure 12: Cystoscope-urethroscope sheath, for examination and irrigation, 7 Fr, with obturator, and 2 LUER-lock connectors

For Use with Deflux Needles

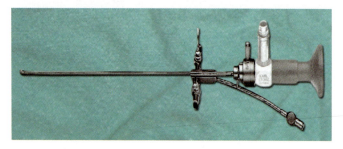

Figure 13: Cystoscope-urethroscope sheath

Cystoscope urethroscope sheath, 8 Fr with 4 Fr working channel, for Deflux needles, with obturator and 2 LUER lock connectors. With the proximally extended working channel in the Deflux sheath, the rigid needles can be gently inserted into the working channel, without becoming blunt (Figures 12 and 13).

Pediatric Resectoscopes

- 9 Fr for use with miniature straight forward telescope (Figures 14A and B).

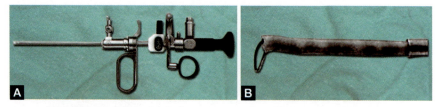

Figures 14A and B: (A) Pediatric resectoscope; (B) Cutting loop–angled

Special features

- Distal end of sheath is atraumatically shaped
- Minimal sheath diameter
- Cutting by means of spring, in rest position, the electrode tip is inside the sheath
- Irrigation possible via HF-connector.

- Resectoscope sheath is 9 Fr with LUER lock stopcock, including connecting tube for inflow.

Pediatric Optical Urethrotome

- 8 Fr for use with miniature straight forward telescope (Figure 15).

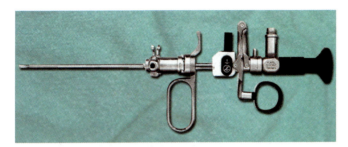

Figure 15: Pediatric optical urethrotome

Special features

- Distal end of sheath is shaped in an atraumatic manner
- Minimal sheath diameter
- Cutting by means of spring, in rest position, the electrode tip is inside the sheath
- Irrigation possible via HF-connector

Urethrotome Sheath with LUER Lock, 8 Fr, with Obturator (Figure 16)

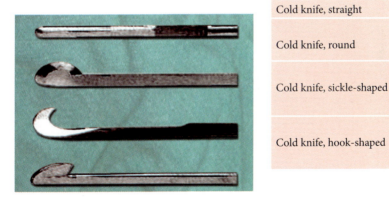

Cold knife, straight
Cold knife, round
Cold knife, sickle-shaped
Cold knife, hook-shaped

Figure 16: Urethrotome sheath with LUER lock, 8 Fr, with obturator

Pediatric Urethrotome (OTIS-KEITZER) (Figure 17)

- OTIS-KEITZER urethrotome, for children, with knife and continuously adjustable from 12 Fr to 30 Fr.

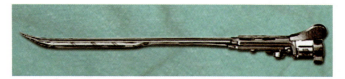

Figure 17: Pediatric urethrotome (OTIS-KEITZER)

Pediatric Percutaneous Nephroscope (Figures 18A and B)

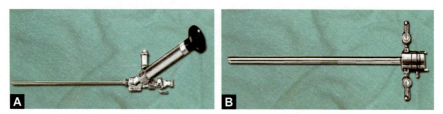

Figures 18A and B: Pediatric percutaneous nephroscope

Hopkins wide angled straight forward telescope 6°, with angled eyepiece, autoclavable, 5 Fr working channel, fiberoptic light transmission is incorporated.

Pediatric Ureterorenoscopes (Figure 19)

• 7.3 Fr, length 25 cm

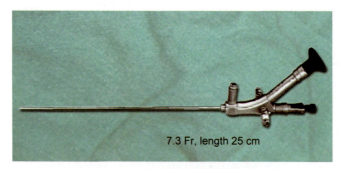

7.3 Fr, length 25 cm

Figure 19: Pediatric ureterorenoscopes

Special features

• Distal tip—7.3 Fr
• Two lateral, right angled irrigation ports
• *Instrument sheath*: 7.3 Fr, conical, 1 step, 7.3 Fr–8 Fr
• *Working channel*: 3.6 Fr for use with instruments up to 3 Fr
• *Telescope*: fiberoptic system, direction of view 6°
• Working length 25 cm.

Index

Page numbers followed by *f* refer to figure and *t* refer to table